Aging Men, Masculinities and Modern Medicine

Aging Men, Masculinities and Modern Medicine explores the multiple socio-historical contexts surrounding men's aging bodies in modern medicine from a global perspective. The first of its kind, it investigates the interrelated aspects of aging, masculinities and biomedicine, allowing for a timely reconsideration of the conceptualization of aging men within the recent explosion of social science studies on men's health and biotechnologies including anti-aging perspectives.

This book discusses both healthy and diseased states of aging men in medical practices, bringing together theoretical and empirical conceptualizations. Divided into four parts it covers:

- Historical epistemology of aging, bodies and masculinity and the way in which the social sciences have theorized the aging body and gender.
- Material practices and processes by which biotechnology, medical assemblages and men's aging bodies relate to concepts of health and illness.
- Aging experience and its impact upon male sexuality and identity.
- The importance of men's roles and identities in care-giving situations and medical practices.

Highlighting how aging men's bodies serve as trajectories for understanding wider issues of masculinity, and the way in which men's social status and men's roles are made in medical cultures, this innovative volume offers a multidisciplinary dialogue between sociology of health and illness, anthropology of the body and gender studies.

Antje Kampf holds a Junior Professorship for the History, Philosophy and Ethics of Medicine (Gender Aspects) at the School of Medicine of the Johannes Gutenberg University Mainz, Germany.

Barbara L. Marshall is Professor of Sociology at Trent University, Canada.

Alan Petersen is Professor of Sociology, School of Political and Social Inquiry, Monash University, Australia.

Routledge Studies in the Sociology of Health and Illness

Available titles include:

Dimensions of Pain
Humanities and social science perspectives
Edited by Lisa Folkmarson Käll

Caring and Well-being
A Lifeworld approach
Kathleen Galvin and Les Todres

Aging Men, Masculinities and Modern Medicine
*Edited by Antje Kampf,
Barbara L. Marshall and Alan Petersen*

Forthcoming titles:

Domestic Violence in Diverse Contexts
A re-examination of gender
Sarah Wendt and Lana Zannettino

Turning Troubles into Problems
Policy and practice in human services
Edited by Jaber F. Gubrium and Margaretha Jarvinen

Aging Men, Masculinities and Modern Medicine

Edited by Antje Kampf,
Barbara L. Marshall and
Alan Petersen

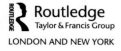

LONDON AND NEW YORK

First published 2013
by Routledge
2 Park Square, Milton Park, Abingdon, Oxon, OX14 4RN

Simultaneously published in the USA and Canada
by Routledge
711 Third Avenue, New York, NY 10017

Routledge is an imprint of the Taylor & Francis Group, an informa business

© 2013 selection and editorial material, Antje Kampf, Barbara L. Marshall and Alan Petersen; individual chapters, the contributors

The right of the editors to be identified as authors of the editorial material, and of the authors for their individual chapters, has been asserted in accordance with sections 77 and 78 of the Copyright, Designs and Patents Act 1988.

All rights reserved. No part of this book may be reprinted or reproduced or utilised in any form or by any electronic, mechanical, or other means, now known or hereafter invented, including photocopying and recording, or in any information storage or retrieval system, without permission in writing from the publishers.

Trademark notice: Product or corporate names may be trademarks or registered trademarks, and are used only for identification and explanation without intent to infringe.

British Library Cataloguing in Publication Data
A catalogue record for this book is available from the British Library

Library of Congress Cataloging in Publication Data
Aging men, masculinities and modern medicine / edited by Antje Kampf, Barbara L. Marshall and Alan Petersen.
    p. cm.
 1. Older men – Health and hygiene. 2. Aging. 3. Masculinity.
 I. Kampf, Antje. II. Marshall, Barbara L. III. Petersen, Alan R., Ph. D.
 RA777.6A37 2013
 613´.04234–dc23   2012019163

ISBN: 978-0-415-69938-9 (hbk)
ISBN: 978-0-203-08137-2 (ebk)

Typeset in Sabon
by HWA Text and Data Management, London

Contents

Notes on contributors vii
Acknowledgements x

Aging men, masculinities and modern medicine:
An introduction 1
ANTJE KAMPF, BARBARA L. MARSHALL AND ALAN PETERSEN

PART I
Rethinking concepts: historical perspectives 19

1 Aging, embodiment and the negotiation of the Third
 and Fourth Ages 21
 PAUL HIGGS AND FIONA MCGOWAN

2 Testosterone and the pharmaceuticalization of male aging 35
 ELIZABETH SIEGEL WATKINS

3 'There is a person here': Rethinking age(ing), gender and
 prostate cancer 52
 ANTJE KAMPF

PART II
Scientific and health discourses on aging men 69

4 Aging men: Resisting and endorsing medicalization 71
 ELIANNE RISKA

5 The vicissitudes of 'healthy aging': The experiences of older
 migrant men in a rural Australian community 86
 SUSAN FELDMAN, ALAN PETERSEN AND HARRIET RADERMACHER

6 What a difference a gay makes: The constitution of the 'older gay man' 105
WILLIAM LEONARD, DUANE DUNCAN AND CATHERINE BARRETT

PART III
Aging, sexualities and identities 121

7 Decreasing erectile function and age-appropriate masculinities in Mexico 123
EMILY WENTZELL

8 Enhancing masculinity and sexuality in later life through modern medicine: Experiences of polygynous Yoruba men in southwest Nigeria 138
AGUNBIADE OJO MELVIN

9 'I haven't died yet': Navigating masculinity, aging and andropause in Turkey 156
MARAL EROL AND CENK ÖZBAY

PART IV
Care work 173

10 Older men: The health and caring paradox 175
KATE DAVIDSON

11 Aging men, masculinity and Alzheimer's: Caretaking and caregiving in the new millennium 191
BETHANY COSTON AND MICHAEL KIMMEL

Index 201

Notes on contributors

Catherine Barrett, PhD, is a Research Fellow and Community Liaison Officer at La Trobe University with a particular focus on sexual health and aging, including GLBTI aging.

Bethany Coston is a PhD candidate at SUNY Stony Brook. She has published in both *Queering Paradigms II*, and the *Journal of Social Issues*. Her current work is on the dynamic processes of power and inequality on violence in heterosexual and queer intimate relationships.

Kate Davidson, PhD, is a Senior Visiting Fellow and co-director of the Centre for Research on Ageing at the University of Surrey, UK. Her research expertise includes qualitative methods examining the lives of older people, focusing on their health and social relationships, especially those of older men.

Duane Duncan, PhD, is a Research Fellow at La Trobe University, Melbourne, Australia, and has published work on gay men, embodiment and sexuality.

Maral Erol, PhD, is a Postdoctoral Fellow at Duke University. Her research interests are gender, science and technology relations with a focus on biomedical technologies and medicalization. She is currently working on discourses related to menopause and the NovaSure procedure.

Susan Feldman, Associate Professor and Director, Healthy Ageing Research Unit, Monash University, is a social gerontologist. Her research interests include the health and well-being of older women, the experience of widowhood, and people from culturally and linguistically diverse communities and relationships between the generations.

Paul Higgs is the Professor of the Sociology of Ageing at University College London. He is the co-author with Ian R. Jones of *Medical Sociology and Old Age* (2009); and with Chris Gilleard of *Cultures of Ageing* (2000) and *Contexts of Ageing* (2005). A third volume on embodiment in aging is due 2013.

Antje Kampf (PhD Auckland, M.A. Cincinnati) holds a Junior Professorship for the History, Philosophy and Ethics of Medicine at the University Medical Center of the Johannes Gutenberg-University Mainz. Her research explores the interrelation of medical cultures of knowledge and representation of aging and gendered bodies.

Michael Kimmel is Distinguished Professor at SUNY Stony Brook. His books include *Manhood in America*, *The Gendered Society*, and *Guyland*.

William Leonard is Director of Gay and Lesbian Health Victoria and has researched and published in the areas of GLBT health and well-being policy and queer theory.

Barbara L. Marshall is Professor of Sociology at Trent University in Peterborough, Canada. Her work explores the intersections of aging, gender, sexuality, bodies and biomedicine. Her current research investigates newly complex discourses and images of a sexualized 'Third Age'.

Fiona McGowan is a Lecturer in Public Health at the University of East London. From a nursing and social care background, she gained her PhD in Medical Sociology at University College London in 2004. Her research focused on the embodiment of masculinity within the context of the life course.

Agunbiade Ojo Melvin is a Lecturer at the Obafemi Awolowo University, Department of Sociology and Anthropology. His ongoing PhD thesis focuses on cultural constructions of sexuality in later life among Yoruba people.

Cenk Özbay is Assistant Professor at Bogazici University in Istanbul, Turkey (PhD in sociology, University of Southern California). He is interested in masculinities, sexualities, class, workplace, neoliberalism, globalization, the city and mobilities. His recent publication is the co-edited volume *Neoliberalizm ve Mahremiyet: Turkiye'de Beden, Saglik ve Cinsellik* (2011).

Alan Petersen is Professor of Sociology, School of Political and Social Inquiry, Monash University in Melbourne, Australia. His research interests span the sociology of health and medicine, science and technology studies, and the construction of sex/gender. His most recent book is *The Politics of Bioethics* (Routledge, 2011). He is currently writing another book, *Hope in Health: The Socio-Politics of Expectations* (Palgrave, forthcoming 2013).

Harriet Radermacher, PhD, is a Research Fellow at the Primary Care Research Unit, Faculty of Medicine, Nursing and Health Sciences Monash University. With a background in Community and Applied Psychology, her research explores the experiences of people marginalized in current society, with a focus on cultural diversity and aging.

Elianne Riska is Professor of Sociology, Vice Rector and Head of Research at the Swedish School of Social Science at the University of Helsinki, Finland.

Elizabeth Siegel Watkins is Dean of the Graduate Division and Professor of History of Health Sciences at the University of California, San Francisco. She is the author of *The Estrogen Elixir: A History of Hormone Replacement Therapy in America* and co-editor of *Prescribed: Writing, Filling, Using, and Abusing the Prescription in Modern America*.

Emily Wentzell is Assistant Professor of Anthropology at the University of Iowa. Her research investigates the social consequences of sexual health intervention in Mexico. Her book *Maturing Machos: Aging and Illness in Post-Viagra Mexico*, is forthcoming from Duke University Press.

Acknowledgements

As always, it's people who make a difference. So, first we would like to thank the contributors of this volume for their fabulous work and wholehearted commitment to our project as it has evolved. Thanks also go to Routledge for their interest and support of our idea, specifically to Grace McInnes and James Watson for their help along the way. We also appreciate the anonymous reviewers for their insightful comments. As a joint project, and an interdisciplinary adventure, working together on this volume has been exceptional.

Antje would like to thank Barbara and Alan for taking the leap and for their dedicated and spot-on comments, criticisms and suggestions. Alan and Barbara would like to thank Antje for her initiative in conceptualizing this volume, her invitation for us to join her in the project, and her hard work in keeping it all on track. It has been no small feat to coordinate the work of three editors on three different continents!

An earlier version of Chapter 11 was published in *The Shriver Report: A Woman's Nation Takes on Alzheimer's* (Washington, DC: Alzheimer's Association, 2010), © 2010 by Michael Kimmel and Bethany Coston. Reprinted by permission. All rights reserved. We are grateful to the American Alzheimer's Association for their permission to publish an extended and revised version of that paper here.

Aging men, masculinities and modern medicine

An introduction

Antje Kampf, Barbara L. Marshall and Alan Petersen

A focus on men's health is a recent concern in both popular and academic literatures. Despite their lower life expectancies and greater susceptibility to major illnesses like heart disease, men have long been viewed as more passive in their attitudes towards help-seeking. Without a clear focus like gynaecology provided for women, institutionalized medicine has tended to marginalize 'men's health' as a specific concern. However, over the last few years, this situation has shifted dramatically, with a notable increase in research and writing on men's health issues.

This new focus on men as a research category has coincided with rapidly increasing aging populations in Western nations, with attendant concerns about the consequences for already-strained health and social service systems. World Health Day in 2012, for example, focused on the theme of aging and health, aiming no less than for a 'need to reinvent aging' (WHO 2012). Since the late 1990s, the 'aging male' in particular has become the focus of an expanding constellation of professional and health promotion concerns. As the mission statement of the International Society for the Study of the Aging Male put it, 'healthy aging and survival of men will have an impact on both family and society. Therefore, the aging of the human male requires special consideration' (1999: 6).

An emphasis on 'healthy', 'positive' and 'active' aging is part of a larger social agenda, linked to neoliberal politics, which encourages risk-averse, self-reliant lifestyles in aging populations (Cardona 2008). The 'Third Age', characterized by independence, healthy lifestyles and activity, is distinguished from the 'Fourth Age' of decrepitude and decline (Gilleard and Higgs 2010, 2011b), and is marked by differences of gender and sexuality across the life course (Marshall and Katz 2006). These differences interact with cultural ageism to shape the ways that men are expected to conform to idealized and youth-based standards of both health and masculinity.

Conceptions of aging men are strongly influenced by scientific explanations of men's corporeal aging (and especially their sexual health) that circulate via diverse media (Hearn 1995). Belief in the potential to delay the process of aging and to enhance the capacities of aging bodies undoubtedly owes much to the growing dominance of the life sciences, specifically biomedicine, in explaining 'life itself' (Rose 2007a). New biomedical technologies (such as biomarkers, enhancement drugs and the rise of anti-ageing or longevity medicine) ground a material turn in understanding men's aging bodies. That is, they reflect a belief in the ability to alter 'natural' processes and even 'turn back the biological clock'. These developments, we contend, call for new approaches to investigate the ways and the extent to which bodies are sites of naturalized political, social and cultural norms and values that serve to shape access to social, economic and political resources.

Though the body is now considered central to any discussion of the political, social and cultural experience of masculinity and masculine identities, this was not the case in early work in the sociology of masculinity, where discussions of men's power and privilege in structural terms tended to predominate (see Petersen 1998, 2007; Applegate 1997). Connell's influential concept of 'hegemonic masculinity' was distinguished from subordinated masculinities, thus drawing attention to gendered power relations *among* men. Critiques of hegemonic masculinity (and by extension the ideal of hetero-normative sexuality) have dominated (and continue to dominate) the development of studies on men's bodies and their experiences with health, illness and medicine. Recent work has brought to the fore hitherto untheorized and unscrutinized aspects of men's bodies, including their pathologization and rehabilitation across a range of contexts (Rosenfeld and Faircloth 2006; Whitehead 2002). This has contributed to a surge of sociologically inspired studies on men's health (e.g. Broom and Tovey 2009; Dolan 2009; Robertson 2007; Courtenay 2000).

It is not that the categories of aging and masculinity have not been analysed together. There is a growing number of studies (e.g. Arber *et al.* 2003), highlighting the changing relations and identities of men and women in later life. Gender theory has become important in gerontological research (Calasanti and Slevin 2006; Calasanti and King 2005; Thompson 2006; Blundo and Bowan 2005). However, most work remains focused on social roles, identities and interaction, leaving epistemological frameworks and men's *bodies* largely unexplored. On the other hand, there are studies that have scrutinized men's bodies but without sustained attention to how aging shapes men's health, masculinity, identity and well-being (but see Oliffe 2009). For example, Rosenfeld and Faircloth (2006) bring the sociology of health and the sociology of the body to bear on the pathologization of men's bodies. Broom and Tovey (2009) discuss the social, political and theoretical underpinnings of men's health. Robertson (2007) focuses on men's views and roles within health care practices and health policy, suggesting psychological and sociological aspects that affect health, with an emphasis on the gendered impact on men's behaviour. Finally, Sabo and Gordon (1995) contextualize masculinities and the experiences of men and health, focusing on psychological and clinical factors on health behaviour. While these studies make an important contribution in conceptualizing the ways in which gendered identities play a vital role in the contexts of health, other lines of analysis, such as the relational character of biomedical disease classifications, therapeutic practices and related technologies, especially in relation to aging, have been largely sidelined and remain under-researched across academic fields. For example, historical analyses of men's bodies, modern medicine and health have only recently begun to specifically explore men's aging as a central analytical tool for reconceiving masculinity (Dinges 2007; Watkins 2007; Hofer 2007; Kampf 2009).

In short, despite the explosion in scholarship on men's bodies and health, the topic of aging men has tended to be neglected. As van den Hoonaard argues, in taking stock of recent developments within critical gerontology and gender studies as a whole, aging and masculinity is 'A topic whose time has come' (2007: 277). The lack of research in this area is perplexing, given both increasing interest in aging culture and its impact upon social and medical systems, and the significance of aging's impact on men's roles and identities.

Overview of the volume

Analytical approach

This collection aims to theorize connections between aging, masculinity, medical practices and knowledge production, thereby contributing to the development of a potentially fertile new field of inquiry. In bringing together research from Mexico, the US, Australia, Germany, Nigeria, Turkey and the UK, the collection offers an international perspective on the socio-historical contexts that shape understandings of and responses to men's aging bodies. We contend that studying constructions of, and responses to, aging men may help reveal wider issues pertaining to masculinity, particularly the processes whereby men's social status and roles are made and understood in the context of biomedical cultures (cf. Marshall 2009; Kampf 2009; Higgs and Jones 2008; Calasanti 2004). Contributors uncover the multiple ways in which bodily knowledge is produced by biomedical technologies and negotiated by aging men themselves. In doing so, they build on a growing body of scholarship that has highlighted the relation between masculinities and aging and the rise of biomedicine and biomedical technologies that are rapidly shaping the meaning of aged health and illness (see e.g. Joyce and Loe 2010; Kampf and Botelho 2009; Kampf 2010; Marshall 2009; Moreira and Palladino 2009). The book offers a multidisciplinary dialogue between the sociology of health and illness, the anthropology of the body, history and gender studies. Premised on the assumption that inquiries into the meaning of the body cannot be approached from a single perspective, the collection, we hope, will prompt a reconceptualization of thinking about men, masculinities and aging.

As recent research emphasizes, there are differences not only between older women and men but also *among* older men (Higgs and Jones 2008).

Moving beyond conceptualizing masculinities solely in terms of inherited power status and hegemony, the chapters draw attention to the vulnerabilities that affect people irrespective of gender (Arber *et al.* 2003). We ground this understanding in current feminist scholarship on the relational processes and practices pertaining to the materiality and embodiment of aging masculinities (Calasanti 2004). Reflecting recent scholarship on the interplay of aging, masculinities and modern medicine, the volume questions the permeability and instability of definitions of aging and gender boundaries within the current politics of health and aging. In their various ways, the authors make reference to the relational practices and materialities involved in the shaping of masculinities, building on earlier work in men's studies (see Petersen 1998; Hearn 2004; Alaimo and Hekman 2008; Connell and Messerschmidt 2005; Kimmel and Aronson 2003). Eschewing binaries of nature/culture, and subject/object (see Haraway 1988; Butler 1993; Bordo 1999), the collection contributes to an interrogation of practices produced by biomedical knowledge about aging men's bodies and health, thus calling into question taken-for-granted categories of disease classification (see also Fujimura 1996; Dumit and Burri 2007). Building on feminist scholars' enquiries into how the body is shaped by and through cultural norms and ideals (Lock and Farquhar 2007; Fausto-Sterling 2005), the chapters highlight the significance of materiality: that is, the conceptualization of men's bodies and practices through embedded and mediated technologies, institutions, and artefacts (Barad 2003).

Framing concepts

Comprising a combination of historical and contemporary scholarship, this collection investigates both healthy and diseased states of aging men, and their relation to biomedical discourses and practices. The chapters raise questions about the implications of different aging experiences, creating a much-needed dialogue about the relationships among bodies/embodiment, technologies and practices. In doing so, they encourage new ways of thinking about and researching biomedical cultures and aging male bodies across disciplines. Bridging theoretical and empirical inquiry, the volume is framed by the following concepts: medicalization/biomedicalization, hegemonic masculinities, the Third Age/Fourth Age distinction and the body/embodiment. All of these concepts are flexible, overlapping and interrelated, and together they orient our understanding of processes of aging and constructions of masculinity in relation to modern biomedicine.

Medicalization/biomedicalization

Many of the cases presented in this collection work with concepts of medicalization and biomedicalization – the latter term emphasizing the increased importance of biomedical technologies of surveillance and treatment (Clarke *et al.* 2003, 2010; Estes and Binney 1989; Kaufman *et al.* 2004). Peter Conrad observes that in the past the literature on gender and medicalization has tended to focus on women 'because their physiological processes (menstruation, birth) are visible, their social roles expose them to medical scrutiny, and they are often in a subordinate position to men in the clinical domain' (2007: 24). However, recent scientific and medical developments, and the emergence of new categories such as 'male menopause' or 'andropause' and 'erectile dysfunction', and new treatments for the aging male body (e.g. testosterone, hair transplants, Viagra) call for a broader understanding of medicalization as a gendered concept (2007: 24–6). Further, Clarke *et al.* note the absence of the explicit problematization and theorization of men's health from a gendered perspective in the early years of study (1970s to 1990s) and 'hardly any *sociological* research on the medicalized character of men's health' (2010: 154; their emphasis). In their view, this trend has now been reversed, with a greater focus on the male body, especially men's sexual health. They see post-structural theory as having contributed to this trend, in that 'men's health has been a means to elaborate the gendered character of knowledge making, to think of gender in relational terms, and to deconstruct binary notions of gender' (2010: 155). Recent scholarship has also encouraged more complex accounts of medicalization (and de-medicalization) which acknowledge multiple and reciprocal processes. As Nikolas Rose suggests, medicalization as a concept might be seen as 'the starting point of an analysis, a sign of the need for analysis, but it should not be the conclusion of an analysis' (2007b: 702; cf. also Clarke *et al.* 2010). With a number of contributions to this collection stemming from outside North America (a focus that has so far dominated scholarly attention, cf. Clarke *et al.* 2010: 39), the contributors are able to unravel the complexity of the emergence of new technologies and disease concepts by illustrating resistance and challenges to (bio)medicalization (e.g. Riska; Feldman *et al.*; Wentzell in this volume).

Hegemonic masculinities

A number of chapters explore changes in the assumed power status of men as they interact with medical discourses and practices as they age. The theme of hegemonic masculinities, while well-travelled in critical men's studies, appears poised to remain for a little longer (cf. also Meadows and Davidson 2006). Ironically, hetero-normativity as a powerful component of hegemonic masculinities has been undertheorized with respect to aging men (but see Duncan and Barrett this volume). The socio-cultural theme of hegemonic masculinities, that carries with it assumptions about the normalization of the male body (and by extension male sexual performance; see also Marshall and Katz 2002) and that can be readily found in medical and socio-cultural scripts of masculinity (see also Moore 2002: 114), seems to have attracted more attention in social science studies investigating the ways in which youth-associated standards of masculinities are potentially *restored*. This has tended to sideline issues related to altered masculinities in the 'Fourth Age' (as described below). The cases presented in this collection come to diverse, even contrary findings about masculinity and men's power. While the contributions by Melvin and Erol and Özbay, for example, reveal strong socio-cultural discourses stabilizing hegemonic masculinity (and hetero-normativity) among aging men, Wentzell's study unravels a resistance by older men to conventional masculine scripts. However, hegemonic masculinities, infused with hetero-normativity, continue to shape health policy and medical practices, and they may fall short in meeting the diversity of men's needs with adverse effects on their well-being (see e.g. Feldman *et al.*; Riska; Watkins; Melvin; Kampf, all in this volume).

The Third Age/Fourth Age distinction

What would effective policy and medical approaches look like? In the introduction to a recent collection on the implications of health promotion and prevention programmes in neoliberal societies, Thomas Mathar and Yvonne Jansen note that 'different forms of knowing the process of ageing inherently transport ethical assumptions because they make claims on what "normal ageing" actually is' (Mathar and Jansen 2010: 23). In fact, articulating what is meant by the condition, process or status of aging is vital when seeking to understand the interrelationships of masculinity and aging in medical contexts. In this collection, we highlight the experiences of 'older men', that is, those inhabiting what have been referred to as the Third and Fourth Ages. The latter is still a very under-researched area, and both 'ages' are still undertheorized and under-researched in their relation to medicine (Higgs and Jones 2008; Flemming 1998). This does not mean that we limit 'aging' to a specific time period or that we understand age to be restricted to pathologies. In fact, it is the other way around: there is still a considerable lack of scholarship engaging theoretically and empirically with the complexity and diversity of men later in their lives. In contrast to assumptions of continuing fitness, vitality and agency in the Third Age (see Carr and Comp 2011), there is a strong association of old age with dependence and decline in physical and mental well-being, impairment and inability to care for one's self and others, and of a loss of meaningful identity. As Gilleard and Higgs argue, we might understand the Fourth Age as 'a kind of social or cultural "black hole" that exercises a powerful gravitational pull upon the surrounding field of aging' (Gilleard and Higgs 2010: 121–2). The Third Age/Fourth Age distinction foregrounds important cultural as well as socio-political issues that need scholarly attention. That 'old age' is a flexible process that might call forth multiple masculinities is evident in a number of the chapters in this volume. Some contributors explicitly address this distinction (e.g. Higgs and McGowan) and explore the implications of a focus on 'healthy' masculine aging in different contexts (e.g. Watkins; Riska).

Others offer specific research rethinking aging men and masculinities in the context of impairment that might come with aging (e.g. Kampf; Davidson; Coston and Kimmel). Clearly, there needs to be more critical discussion of these issues as current demands on health and welfare systems and individuals negotiating them have to come to terms with both extended life spans and the challenges of chronic diseases and conditions.

The body/embodiment

Finally, *Aging Men, Masculinities and Modern Medicine* emphasizes the body and embodiment as central to the definition and experience of aging. Considering and giving room to the body and embodied experiences and identities is vital if we are to understand the relationships among masculinity, aging, healthiness and disease (Featherstone and Hepworth 1998; Gilleard and Higgs 2011a; Hockey and James 2004; Katz 2011; Laz, 2003; Twigg 2004; Watson 2000). Such a focus is particularly important when considered in conjunction with the recent emphasis in health promotion on self-care and on taking control of one's health and body (see e.g. Ziguras 2004). We do not elaborate on the complexity of this turn to 'behaviour' here (but see e.g. Armstrong 2009). However, in contrast to the focus in health economics and epidemiology on aggregate data, or bio-political concerns with managing aging, ailing bodies, our contributors provide rich insights into experiences of embodiment by aging men in diverse contexts. Here, men's *physical* experience of growing older is considered in contexts that include varying expressions of hegemonic masculinities and the spectre of the Fourth Age in undoing them. In doing so, they add important insights to growing strands of scholarship exploring the body and embodiment in relation to masculinities, aging and medical cultures that have to date largely proceed in isolation from one another.

Overview of the chapters

The volume is divided into four sections, each of which engages with these concepts in varying interrelated ways.

Part I, 'Rethinking concepts: historical perspectives', focuses on historical epistemologies of aging, bodies and masculinity and the ways in which the social sciences have theorized the aging body and gender. The chapters in this section tackle the major concepts discussed earlier and while they can stand on their own, they can equally offer a theoretical and historical contextualization as an entry point from which one can read the subsequent sections.

The first paper in this section, by Paul Higgs and Fiona McGowan, develops the theme of changing conceptions of aging and masculinity. Drawing on theories of 'second modernity' (Beck) with its individualization of life courses and emphasis on agency, choice and consumption, they argue that conventional assumptions about age, bodies and masculinity have been 'radically disturbed'. The Third Age is conceptualized as a cultural field that frames a new emphasis on continued performance of masculine identity into later life, dependent on maintaining bodily fitness and vitality. Aging men have become an important and growing market for pharmaceutical and biotechnical products, especially those that promise to restore sexual virility, and by proxy, the very masculinity that aging threatens. The agentic, active Third Age can only be fully understood in relation to the powerful imaginary of the Fourth Age of decline and decrepitude, where 'the capacity to perform any sort of masculinity is impossible'. In mapping out the embodied nature of the distinction between the Third and Fourth Ages, Higgs and McGowan provide an indispensable overview of the cultural landscape that shapes contemporary masculine encounters with medicine and the discourses of 'health' and 'fitness'.

Elizabeth Watkins's chapter provides an exemplary case of how aging and masculinities are configured historically in relation to biomedical and commercial interests – highlighting specifically the Third Age. Focusing on the separation of low testosterone from normal aging and the proposal of a pharmaceutical solution, Watkins reminds us that testosterone has a history, initially synthesized in the 1930s, taken up (though not uniformly) by mainstream medicine in 1940s, and largely abandoned by the 1950s. Watkins tackles the question of why, after years of neglect, notions of a hormonally treatable male menopause were revived in the 1990s, and how the framing of this 'disorder' has evolved. Her analysis highlights both shifts in cultural understandings of masculinity, aging and health and an intensified 'reductionism' in medicine that favours quantitative indicators of disease states. Focusing on the 'medical-industrial complex', she shows that there was a range of 'mutually reinforcing' developments in science, biotechnology, clinical practice and pharmaceutical marketing that produced what is now known as 'Low T' – a quantitatively identifiable condition affecting aging men, linked to a readily available pharmaceutical treatment. As she concludes, 'medicalization, pharmaceuticalization and commercialization occurred within an assemblage of changing roles for men as health care consumers ... changing definitions and performances of masculinities and changing expectations for medicine and pharmaceuticals in preventing diseases associated with growing old'.

In the final paper in this section, Antje Kampf develops the themes of embodiment, materiality and masculinity as they intersect with medical discourses through the example of prostate cancer. Kampf draws on feminist theories of embodiment and corporeality in her exploration of the production of discourses around prostate cancer – including biomedical technologies of diagnosis, treatment and risk management. Drawing on historical and contemporary clinical literature, as well as men's own narratives in online forums on prostate cancer, Kampf teases out the different configurations of masculine bodies that emerge within social science scholarship. These include the aging body, the sexual body, the statistical body and the social body, each of which provides a lens for understanding 'how bodies are lived in and shaped, how they are technically mediated and how they are experienced'. Like Watkins, she reveals a history to the development of a disease entity that is complex, sometimes contradictory, and reflects cultural shifts in understandings of masculinity, aging and health. Kampf emphasizes the ways in which aging male bodies are materialized in prostate cancer discourses, and calls for more attention to the *social* bodies of aging men in future research.

The chapters in Part II, 'Scientific and health discourses on aging men', tackle the ways in which biotechnology, medical diagnoses and practices and men's aging bodies produce and are produced by, relate to, negotiate and define health and illness. Included here is analysis and reconsideration of concepts of hetero-normativity, and related (and contested) constructions of medicalization processes and health care provision.

Elianne Riska's paper argues that medicalization has proceeded in different ways for men and women, with traditional 'sex-role' theory still more evident in shaping the conceptualization of men's health in public health discourse. As she describes it, this approach treats men's health behaviours as 'cultural affirmation of the masculine script' and risks naturalizing men's health and bodies. She critically engages with the implications of this through examining two scientific discourses on men's health that demonstrate men's resistance to, and endorsement of, a medicalization of aging: (1) post traumatic stress disorder (PTSD) as a psychiatric diagnosis of aging war veterans' mental health issues, and (2) androgen deficiency (and the related diagnoses of testosterone deficiency syndrome (TDS) and erectile dysfunction (ED)). While both of these encapsulate aspects of de-masculinization according to conventional scripts, they differ in the ways they have been taken up by affected men. The discourse of PTSD, Riska suggests, has resulted in challenges and resistance to the 'pathologization of failed masculinity' that such medicalization implies. Men's tacit acceptance of the endocrinologically constituted male body offered in the discourse of TDS/ED, on the other hand, is illustrative of *bio*medicalization, where the 'interactions of technoscience, biomedical professionals and pharmaceutical corporations' are authorized to 'produce a definition of a deviation from the norm and a pathologization of that deviation'.

Susan Feldman, Alan Petersen and Harriet Radermacher shift the focus to the ways in which the experiences of older men from culturally and linguistically diverse (CALD) backgrounds challenge dominant biomedical perspectives on aging. Based on fieldwork in rural Australia with both older men and health care providers, their chapter provides compelling evidence that the biomedical focus on illness, decline and universalized interventions to correct dysfunctions in aging men (especially sexual dysfunctions) is inadequate in addressing the health needs of a diverse population of aging men. They explore the ways in which age, ethnicity, gender and rural location intersect in ways that underscore the futility of one-size-fits-all models of 'aging males' and their health needs. Unsettling the biomedical conception of aging and its focus on 'the biophysical body and processes of physical and mental decline', this chapter suggests a substantial rethinking of how 'healthy aging' might be conceptualized in relation to men. For example, a key theme emerging from their research is the desire of older men to maintain their sense of independence, identity, control and connectedness to family and community. As they conclude, 'understanding the socio-cultural shaping and complexity of experiences of health and well-being is essential if healthcare interventions are to be effective'.

In a similar vein, William Leonard, Duane Duncan and Catherine Barrett argue that the narrow focus on gender in men's health diverts attention away from the most pressing needs of aging men. Such is the case, they argue, when looking at the process of marginalizing the experiences of gay men. Leonard et al. seek to address this gap, focusing on how gay male embodiment, masculinity and aging have been shaped by a range of biomedical and social technologies. They explore masculinity as a heterosexual construct and review the ways in which gay identity emerged in concert with medicalized conceptions of the body in the late twentieth century. In particular, the emergence of HIV/AIDS as a 'gay disease' in the 1980s and 1990s constituted gay men's bodies as particular sites of social concern and anxiety. Historically, such discourses have also positioned gay men in a paradoxical relationship to orthodox masculinities. The emergence of new biotechnologies and the increasing medicalization of aging offers men – both gay and heterosexual – new practices and potential identities that both reinforce and reshape traditional ideas about masculinity (as has been also highlighted by Riska). Leonard et al. note that while, on the one hand, there are increasing parallels between the experiences of aging gay and heterosexual men, on the other hand, biomedical technologies and forms of heath care organization threaten to shore up hetero-normative masculinities and reassert negative stereotypes of gay men. Reviewing a range of qualitative research with aging gay men, this chapter illustrates the complex ways in which contemporary practices of sexuality, masculinity and medicine intersect, and the manner in which homophobia continues to shape older gay men's sense of masculinity and embodiment.

In Part III, 'Aging, sexualities and identities', the chapters engage with the impact and extent of cultural assumptions about masculinity, particularly sexuality, on aging men's health and concepts of identity. Importantly, they draw attention to the way in which aging men make sense of these cultural constructions in diverse settings, revealing that the idealized concept of hegemonic masculinities can lead to very different outcomes for aging men in their local situations.

Emily Wentzell's paper contextualizes the issue of erectile dysfunction (ED) and challenges to hegemonic masculinities as these have played out in Mexico, where stereotypic notions of 'macho' masculinity provide a powerful framework for individual biographies. Based on interviews with 250 mostly working-class men seeking treatment from the urology department of an urban, public hospital, Wentzell's research provides a fascinating picture of constructions of age, sexuality and masculinized masculinities that unsettles assumptions about their universality or transferability across cultural contexts. As she notes, 'people relate to drugs like Viagra in locally-specific ways'. Unlike the Yoruba men discussed by Melvin in the chapter which follows, the older men interviewed by Wentzell rejected the notion that decreasing erectile function in later life was pathological, and this led them to resist medicalization and pharmaceutical solutions. Her chapter describes in detail the story of 'Jorge', an 82-year-old testicular amputee, as an example to illustrate how older men may not only accept decreasing erectile function as a normal consequence of aging, but may incorporate decreasing sexual function into their conceptions and practices of 'good' older masculinity. Jorge, alongside Wentzell's other participants, 'present a reminder that biomedicine is a cultural system, used in contexts where definitions of a healthy sex life are shaped by local ideals about gender, aging, sex and love'.

Like Wentzell, Agunbiade Ojo Melvin also draws on research with both older men and health care providers but the setting here is urban Nigeria with a focus on their conceptions of *sexually* aging well. Aging men in this context accept aspects of medicalization and use modern heath care services, but at the same time maintain traditional cultural constructions of what it means to 'age well'. Melvin interviewed both polygamous Yoruba men aged 50–75 and health care providers (physicians and nurses), and finds variations in the experiences of the former and the perceptions of the latter. Interviews with men revealed deeply rooted conceptions of masculinity that centre sexual prowess and virility across the life course. They interpreted the need to constantly satisfy their wives sexually as requiring medical intervention as they age. Health care providers tended to emphasize cultural constructs of 'exemplary adults' by arguing that sexually aging might well entail de-emphasizing sex, and embracing the social responsibilities (such as grand-fatherhood) that accompany aging. Thus, the use of medical technology for enhancing (or maintaining) sexuality did not always proceed smoothly, nor was modern medicine the panacea for all their needs, as 'unofficial' remedies also proliferated. The context explored here provides a unique lens for viewing the intersections of modern medicine with local constructions of aging male bodies.

Maral Erol and Cenk Özbay explore an emerging discourse on medicalized (and sexualized) aging masculinities in Turkey, where 'public debate about masculinity is yet to be matured and stabilized'. Already-accepted trajectories of female bodily aging (menopause) offered a medicalized language to describe male anxieties about aging and the issues faced by middle-aged heterosexual couples (andropause). However, the ways in which this has been taken up have varied. Erol and Özbay analyse coverage of 'andropause' in the Turkish press over a ten-year period, identifying three distinct strands of debates about the hormonal model of aging male bodies: (1) andropause as a medical problem, with attendant concerns about prevention and treatment, (2) andropause as a social problem, where it is viewed as an 'excuse for marital infidelity', and (3) andropause as an 'insult', deployed to suggest unsuccessful negotiation of a 'midlife crisis', and used to demean political rivals. Thus, while the construction of women's menopause has treated it as universal and inevitable, and has thus tended to assume women's increased responsibility for self-care and healthy decision-making, the same is not true of andropause. The 'health-related obligation of seeking medical help and surveillance ... in the andropause narratives of health columns and interviews with doctors' competes with counter-discourses of 'horny goats' and midlife crises that scold aging men, yet are ultimately tolerant of hegemonic masculinities.

Part IV, 'Care Work', traces aging experience and individual life worlds – the 'orphan child of the scientized world' (Beck 1995: 15) – as they configure (and are configured by) men's roles and identities in care-giving situations, medical practices and social and cultural discourses more broadly. The papers in this concluding section bring the collection full circle, turning to this under-researched but important aspect of the Fourth Age.

Kate Davidson finds that, despite increased experience of physical frailties as their aging bodies 'let them down', many older men call 'on their sense of manhood, resilience and stoicism to negotiate and define their experience of aging'. Her chapter demonstrates the trials and tribulations of older men as they deal with failing health and illness; bodily states that might indicate the Fourth Age as described by Higgs and McGowan. While these might be seen as a threat to their perceived masculine ideals, they may motivate men to pay attention to their bodies in order to resist this, and maintain employment status, pursue sporting activities and/or care for family members. Thus, the care work of older men must be considered in relation to both the care of their own bodies and their care for family members/loved ones. To explore these issues, Davidson draws on her extensive qualitative research in the UK with older men living independently in the community. She argues that, while the men's sense of manhood was undiminished regardless of their physical condition, they applied a 'best fit' attitude to their current embodied experience – what she terms an 'elasticity employed in coming to terms with altered masculine identities'. In doing so, she demonstrates the ways in which masculinity structures men's experiences across the life course, despite the onset of infirmities and/or changes in partnership status. As her conclusions suggest, effective health promotion should move beyond targeting individuals to take into account the broader social determinants of older men's health.

Finally, Bethany Coston and Michael Kimmel also attend to the under-researched topic of older men and care work, but with a focus on mental health. Their focus is on older men as providers – or recipients – of Alzheimer's care in the context of the US, where an aging population has made dementia a major public health concern. Coston and Kimmel enquire into the relationship of masculinity and care work, exploring how traditional definitions of masculinity may inhibit or facilitate men's experiences. With both giving and receiving care traditionally seen as 'feminine', they argue that traditional conceptions of masculinity have ill-prepared men for caregiving, and have shaped their experience of receiving care as potentially de-masculinizing. Alzheimer's, they suggest, may be 'especially difficult to reconcile with traditional notions of masculinity that stress autonomy and control'. However, Coston and Kimmel suggest that there may be generational differences between the current cohort of male Alzheimer's patients and caregivers and those of the future (who have matured in an arguably less rigidly gender-defined culture with respect to caring).

Thinking ahead: developing a research agenda

Taken together, the contributions to *Aging Men, Masculinities and Modern Medicine* offer current research on aging men and masculinity within medicine and medical cultures from an international perspective, illustrating how diverse or indeed similar aging masculinities are defined, enacted and experienced. However, the collection maps out a relatively new field of inquiry, and some key areas of research are only now developing, leaving gaps in what is covered here. These include the ways in which concepts of healthy aging are shaped by racial, class and hetero-normative discourses that are often embedded within biomedicine (Clarke *et al.* 2010: 28–30, 219–30). For example, recent biomedical discourse has tended to conflate the 'healthy ageing' of men with their continued (hetero)sexual virility (Marshall 2009, 2011) and this has prompted a focus in critical scholarship (evident in this volume) on disease entities as such as erectile dysfunction and andropause/low testosterone. There is a need for more research on areas less well covered, including disease conditions, such as heart disease (for an exception, see Riska 2006), diabetes and mental health (but see Kimmel and Coston in this volume), but also on issues related to social and cultural roles, including fatherhood and family relations, and in some cases, social isolation. Certainly more work is required which casts a critical eye on the exclusions produced by biomedical discourse. Biomedicalization has tended to narrow the focus of enquiries, with dominant assumptions about naturalized difference serving to decontexualize disease and illness. The health promotion and policy implications of recent media and medical interest in the 'problem' of failing health in aging men remain underanalysed when it comes to challenging hegemonic masculine scripts. A bias in perspectives on men's health towards changing individual behaviours and providing more 'targeted' services can divert attention from the social structures and practices reinforcing hegemonic masculinity, including those associated with biomedicine. Attention to the full range of issues that shape embodiment, masculinity and encounters with medical discourses and practices in later life – including the 'oldest' old – will provide rich opportunities for analyses that can work with important social dimensions of difference and inequality. Finally, research on aging masculinities will be enhanced through a more global perspective, taking into account not only cultural and political diversity in the contexts of aging, but the local impacts of globalized biomedicine and pharmaceutical culture.

We hope that the papers here provide a catalyst for further work on aging masculinities, which does not conflate masculinity with youth, and which tackles some of the critical questions prompted by considering the ways in which medical discourses and practices shape modern life courses. We will not be able to provide a definite answer as to what it means to grow old as a man in a 'man's body', but we hope that this volume will encourage scholars to invest their time and resources into future endeavours in this important field of inquiry.

References

Alaimo, S., and Hekman, S. (eds) (2008) *Material Feminisms*, Bloomington, IN: Indiana University Press.
Applegate, J. S. (1997) 'Theorizing older men', in J. I. Kosberg and L. W. Kaye (eds), *Elderly Men: Social Problems and Professional Challenges,* (pp. 1–15), New York: Springer.
Arber, S., Davidson, K., and Ginn, J. (eds) (2003) *Gender and Ageing: Changing Roles and Relationships,* Maidenhead: Open University Press.
Armstrong, D. (2009) 'Origins of the problem of health-related behaviours: A genealogical study', *Social Studies of Science*, 39(6): 909–26.
Barad, K. (2003) 'Posthumanist performativity: Toward an understanding of how matter comes to matter', *Signs: Journal of Women in Culture and Society*, 28(3): 801–31.
Beck, U. (1992) *Risk Society: Towards a New Modernity*, London: Sage.
Blundo, R. D., and Bowen, E. (2005) 'Aging and older men: Thoughts, reflections and issues. Introduction', *Journal of Sociology and Social Welfare*, 32(1): 3–7.
Bordo, S. (1999) *The Male Body: A New Look at Men in Public and Private*, New York: Farrar, Straus & Giroux.
Broom, A., and Tovey, P. (eds) (2009) *Men's Health: Body, Identity and Social Context*, London: Wiley.
Butler, J. (1993) *Bodies that Matter: On the Discursive Limits of 'Sex'*, London: Routledge.
Calasanti, T. (2004) 'Feminist gerontology and old men', *Journal of Gerontology: Social Sciences*, 59: S305–S314.
Calasanti, T., and King, N. (2005) 'Firming the floppy penis: Age, class, and gender relations in the lives of old men', *Men and Masculinities,* 8: 3–23.
Calasanti, T., and Slevin, K. F. (eds) (2006) *Age Matters: Re-aligning Feminist Thinking*, New York: Routledge.
Cardona, B. (2008) '"Healthy ageing" policies and anti-ageing ideologies and practices: On the exercise of responsibility', *Medicine, Health Care and Philosophy*, 11(4): 475–83.

Carr, D., and Comp, K. (eds) (2011) *Gerontology in the Era of the Third Age*, New York: Springer.
Clarke, A., Shim, J. K., Mamo, L., Fosket, J. R., and Fishman, J. (2003) 'Biomedicalization: Technoscientific transformations of health, illness and U.S. biomedicine', *American Sociological Review*, 68(2): 161–94.
Clarke, A. E., Mamo, L., Fosket, J. R., Fishman, J. R., and Shim, J. K. (eds) (2010) *Biomedicalization: Technoscience, Health and Illness in the US*, Durham, NC, and London: Duke University Press.
Connell, R., and Messerschmidt, J. W. (2005) 'Hegemonic masculinity: Rethinking the concept', *Gender and Society*, 19(5): 597–623.
Conrad, P. (2007) *The Medicalization of Society: On the Transformation of Human Conditions into Treatable Disorders*, Baltimore, MD: John Hopkins University Press.
Courtenay, W. H. (2000) 'Constructions of masculinity and their influence on men's well-being: A theory of gender and health', *Social Science and Medicine*, 50: 1385–1401.
Dinges, M. (2008) *Männlichkeit und Gesundheit: Im historischen Wandel 1650–2000*, Stuttgart: Steiner.
Dolan, A. (2009) *Men and their Health: Masculinity, Social Inequality and Health (Critical Studies in Health and Society)*, London: Routledge.
Dumit, R. V., and Burri J. (2007) *Biomedicine as Culture: Instrumental Practices, Technoscientific Knowledge, and New Modes of Life*, London: Routledge.
Estes, C., and Binney, E. (1989) 'The biomedicalization of aging: Dangers and dilemmas', *The Gerontologist*, 29(5): 587–96.
Fausto-Sterling, A. (2005) 'The bare bones of sex: Part I, sex and gender', *Signs: Journal of Women in Culture and Society*, 30(2): 1491–1528.
Featherstone, M., and Hepworth, M. (1998) 'Ageing, the lifecourse and the sociology of embodiment', in G. Scambler and P. Higgs (eds), *Modernity, Medicine and Health* (pp.147–75), London: Routledge.
Fujimura, J. H. (1996) *Crafting Science: A Sociohistory of the Quest for the Genetics of Cancer*, Cambridge, MA: Harvard University Press.
Flemming, A. A. (1998) 'Older men in contemporary discourses on aging: Absent bodies and invisible lives', *Nursing Inquiry*, 6(1): 3–8.
Gilleard, C., and Higgs, P. (2010) 'Aging without agency: Theorizing the Fourth Age', *Aging and Mental Health*, 14(2): 121–8.
Gilleard, C., and Higgs, P. (2011a) 'Ageing abjection and embodiment in the Fourth Age', *Journal of Aging Studies*, 25(2): 135–42.
Gilleard, C., and Higgs, P. (2011b) 'The Third Age as a cultural field', in D. C. Carr and K. Komp (eds), *Gerontology in the Era of the Third Age* (pp. 33–49), New York: Springer.
Haraway, D. (1988) 'Situated knowledges: The science question in feminism and the privilege of partial perspective', *Feminist Studies*, 14(3): 577–99.
Hearn, J. (1995) 'Imaging the aging of men', in M. Featherstone and A. Wernick (eds), *Images of Aging: Cultural Representations of Later Life* (pp. 97–115), London: Routledge.
Hearn, J. (2004) 'From hegemonic masculinity to the hegemony of men', *Feminist Theory*, 5: 97–120.
Higgs, P., and Jones, I. R. (2008) *Medical Sociology and Old Age: Towards a Sociology of Health in Later Life*, London: Routledge.

Hockey, J., and James, A. (2004) 'How do we know that we are aging? Embodiment, agency and later life', in E. Tulle (ed.), *Old Age and Agency* (pp. 157–72), New York: Nova Science Publishers.

Hofer, H. G. (2007) 'Climacterium virile, andropause, PADAM: Zur geschichte der männlichen wechseljahre im 20 jahrhundert', in M. Dinges (ed.), *Männlichkeit und Gesundheit: Im historischen Wandel 1650–2000* (pp. 123–38), Stuttgart: Steiner.

International Society for the Study of the Aging Male (1999) 'Mission statement', *The Aging Male*, 2(1): 6–7.

Joyce, K., and Loe, M. (2010) 'A sociological approach to ageing, technology and health', *Sociology of Health and Illness*, 32(2): 171–80.

Kampf, A. (2009) 'The absence of Adam: Prostate cancer and male identity', in J. Powell and T. Gilbert (eds), *Aging and Identity: A Postmodern Dialogue* (pp. 29–43), New York: Nova Science Publishers.

Kampf, A. (2010) '"The risk of age"? Early detection test, prostate cancer and technologies of self', *Journal of Aging Studies*, 24(4): 325–34.

Kampf, A., and Botelho, L. (eds) (2009) 'Special issue: Anti-aging and biomedicine: bodies, gender, and the pursuit of longevity', *Medicine Studies: An International Journal for History, Philosophy, and Ethics of Medicine and Allied Sciences*, 1(3).

Katz, S. (2011) 'Hold on! Falling, embodiment and the materiality of old age', in M. J. Casper and P. Currah (eds), *Corpus: An Interdisciplinary Reader on Bodies and Knowledge* (pp. 187–206), London: Palgrave Macmillan.

Kaufman, S. R., Shim, J. K., and Russ, A. J. (2004) 'Revisiting the biomedicalization of aging: Clinical trends and ethical challenges', *The Gerontologist*, 44(6): 731–8.

Kimmel, M., and Aronson, A. (eds) (2003) *Men and Masculinities: A Social, Cultural, and Historical Encyclopedia*, Santa Barbara, CA: ABC-CLIO-Press.

Laz, C. (2003) 'Age embodied', *Journal of Aging Studies*, 17(4): 503–19.

Lock, M., and J. Farquhar (2007) *Beyond the Body Proper: Reading the Anthropology of Material Life*, Durham, NC: Duke University Press.

Marshall, B. L. (2009) 'Rejuvenation's return: Anti-aging and re-masculinization in biomedical discourse on the "aging male"', *Medicine Studies*, 1(3): 249–65.

Marshall, B. L. (2011) 'The graying of "sexual health": A critical research agenda', *Canadian Review of Sociology*, 48(4): 390–413.

Marshall, B. L., and Katz, S. (2002) 'Forever functional: Sexual fitness and the ageing male body', *Body and Society*, 8(4): 43–70.

Marshall, B. L., and Katz, S. (2006) 'From androgyny to androgens: Re-sexing the aging body', in T. Calasanti and K. Slevin (eds), *Age Matters* (pp. 75–98), New York: Routledge.

Mathar, T., and Jansen, Y. (eds) (2010) *Health, Promotion and Prevention Programmes in Practice*, Bielefeld: Transcript Verlag.

Meadows, R., and Davidson, K. (2006) 'Maintaining manliness in later life: Hegemonic masculinities and emphasized femininities', in T. C. Calasanti and K. F. Slevin (eds), *Age Matters: Realigning Feminist Thinking* (pp. 295–312), New York: Routledge.

Moore, L. J. (2002) 'Extracting men from semen: masculinity in scientific representation of sperm', *Social Text*, 20(4): 91–119.

Moreira, T., and Palladino, P. (2009) 'Ageing between gerontology and biomedicine', *Biosocieties*, 4(4): 348–65.

Oliffe, J. (2009) 'Health behaviors, prostate cancer, and masculinities: A life course perspective', *Men and Masculinities*, 11: 346–66.
Petersen, A. (1998) *Unmasking the Masculine: 'Men' and 'Identity' in a Sceptical Age*, London: Sage.
Petersen, A. (2007) *The Body in Question: A Socio-Cultural Approach*, New York: Routledge.
Powell, J. L., and Gilbert, T. (2009) *Aging and Identity: A Postmodern Dialogue*, New York: Nova Science Publishers.
Riska, E. (2006) *Masculinity and Men's Health: Coronary Heart Disease in Medical and Public Discourse*, New York: Rowman & Littlefield.
Robertson, S. (2007) *Understanding Men's Health: Masculinity, Identity and Well-Being*, Buckingham: Open University Press.
Rose, N. (2007a) *The Politics of Life Itself: Biomedicine, Power, and Subjectivity in the Twenty-First Century*, Princeton, NJ: Princeton University Press.
Rose, N. (2007b) 'Beyond Medicalization', *The Lancet*, 369(9562): 651–714.
Rosenfeld, D., and Faircloth, C. A. (eds) (2006) *Medicalized Masculinities*, Philadelphia, PA: Temple University Press.
Sabo, D. , and Gordon, D. F. (1995) *Men's Health and Illness: Gender, Power, and the Body*, London: Sage.
Thompson, E. H., Jr.(2006) 'Images of old men's masculinity: Still a man?', *Sex Roles*, 55: 633–48.
Thompson, E. H., Jr., and Whearty, P. M. (2004) 'Older men's social participation: The importance of masculinity ideology', *Journal of Men's Studies*, 13(1): 5–24.
Twigg, J. (2004) 'The body, gender and age: Feminist insights in social gerontology', *Journal of Aging Studies*, 18(1): 59–73.
van den Hoonaard, D. B. (2007) 'Aging and masculinity: A topic whose time has come', *Journal of Aging Studies*, 21(4): 277–80.
Watson, J. (2000) *Male Bodies. Health, Culture and Identity*, Buckingham: Open University Press.
Watkins, E. (2007) 'The medicalisation of male menopause in America', *Social History of Medicine*, 20(2): 369–88.
WHO (2012). World Health Day: http://www.who.int/mediacentre/events/annual/world_health_day/en/index.html (accessed April 2012).
Whitehead, S. M (2002) *Men and Masculinities: Key Themes and New Directions*, Oxford: Blackwell.
Ziguras, C. (2004) *Self-Care: Embodiment, Personal Autonomy and the Shaping of Health Consciousness*, London: Routledge.

Part I
Rethinking concepts
Historical perspectives

1 Aging, embodiment and the negotiation of the Third and Fourth Ages

Paul Higgs and Fiona McGowan

It has been widely noted that concerns about the body and embodiment have moved from being primarily focused around women's corporeality to becoming one of the contemporary arenas where masculinity is constructed and performed. This is ever more evident in a society focused around youth and vitality where men are increasingly expected to demonstrate certain levels of health and fitness in the context of narratives of idealized masculine physicality. The issues surrounding age and aging therefore need to be included in any discussion of how masculinity and embodiment interact, and how this relates to medicine and medicalization. Consequently, while biographical and social factors have been found to be significant in shaping and constraining the ways in which men experience the aging process, these factors are not static. Different issues concerning the body, health and the self emerge for men at different points in their lives and these in turn need to be related to the emergence of concepts such as the Third and Fourth Ages. They also need to be related to the role that biomedicine plays in changing the context in which 'aspirational medicine' (Gilleard and Higgs 2000: 187) operates to provide a narrative of enhancement in relation to the aging process. Such enhancements change the nature of 'normative' expectations about later life and as we shall see have a key significance in the negotiation of current forms of masculinity. To date most published work on the significance of aging in constructing the discourses of masculinity and embodiment has underplayed these critical concepts and the way in which they reflect profound changes to what constitutes aging and later life.

This chapter seeks to rectify this omission by drawing attention to changes in the experience of aging by challenging some of the assumptions about the 'natural' nature of the life course and how it refracts male embodiment and ideas of masculinity. In particular, the transformation of the notion of the 'standardized' life course into one that is now more 'de-standardized' (Gilleard and Higgs 2005) is one that has accompanied the transformation of classical modernity into what has been termed 'reflexive modernization' or, in Ulrich Beck's formulation, second modernity (Beck *et al.* 2003). This transformation is particularly noticeable at older ages where the conventional construction of retirement as old age and dependency has been rearticulated through the cultural field of the Third Age (Gilleard and Higgs 2011a). Within the culture of the Third Age, discourses of individuals being older but not old have emerged out of the narratives of a maturing youth culture operating within a burgeoning domain of lifestyle consumption. This cultural domain also resonates with the changing nature of biomedicine which increasingly sees opportunities for enhancement and not just the amelioration of decline. The processes of an aging youth culture and lifestyle consumption therefore make up two vectors of a new 'generational field' of aging in which choice, agency, autonomy and freedom are valorized. In this a gendered bodily dimension becomes apparent with men facing issues of capacity, fitness and virility as challenges as well as the more conventional threats associated with being identified with an older status. These threats exist in direct proportion to individuals' capacity to maintain themselves as active participants in the culture of the Third Age. Consequently, it is not at all surprising that it also leads to an engagement with a range of differentiated anti-aging and self-enhancement technologies which all relate to each individual having to deal with what Higgs and Jones (2009) have termed the 'arc of acquiescence' as they attempt to negotiate the signs and effects of their own bodily aging. For both women and men this engagement may range variously from hair dye to cosmetic surgery as well as extending from vitamin supplements to performance-enhancing pharmaceutical products (Leontowitsch *et al.* 2010). For men while there may be more scope for negotiating a 'mature' image, issues of potency and virility add to the mix (Loe 2006).

Dealing with the pressures created by the agentic culture of the Third Age also means having to face up to its shadow: the Fourth Age. Many writers are reluctant to grapple with this 'dark' side of contemporary aging because it seems to describe later life as one defined by 'lack' and frailty (Grenier 2007). However as Gilleard and Higgs (2010) point out the Fourth Age serves as a powerful 'social imaginary' containing many of the notions of frailty, physical dependency and mental infirmity that most undermine the capacities of adult human actors particularly around agency and identity. Not only is it a position that most would wish to avoid given its unpleasant underpinnings, it is also one from which there seems to be no possibility of escape (Gilleard and Higgs 2011b). In this the Fourth Age throws up specific issues for men and for masculinity as the implicit dependency reverses previously existing power relationships and social boundaries around the body and the care of the body. Given the importance of these two critical dimensions to aging, how men negotiate the Third and Fourth Ages is crucial for the understanding of male embodiment and masculinity in contemporary societies.

Masculinity, youthfulness and the body

Men as much as women are now subject to social expectations in respect of their physical appearance, influenced by the growth of consumer culture where idealized male bodies have become more visible in representing an increasingly dominant and desirable masculinity. A masculine physique has become a symbol of masculinity and as such is valued not so much because of what it can do but because of how it looks. Therefore men with bodies that epitomize hegemonic masculinity and match the cultural ideal – lean, muscular and youthful – have the physical capital most valued in the field of masculinity (Coles 2009). If these embodied qualities of youth are viewed as 'essentially masculine' then aging and old age are the negation of that ideal, threatening men as they age with the obvious failure of matching up to such representations of maleness. Men who were once secure in their body image are now subject to fears of personal devaluation (Whitehead 2002). That this is an ever-present issue can be seen in what Watson (2000: 96) terms 'backward glancing', where middle-aged men look back to their own younger selves in order to sustain their present self-identities. It is this 'idealized image' of the young fit body which is retained by the older man and it continues to contribute to the masculine sense of self as men grow older and age. This active yet 'dated' image is 'attached to current masculine identity' and helps explain men's reluctance to acknowledge bodily changes regarded as intrinsically negative. Growing older therefore requires men to renegotiate masculine identities and just as the body is transformed through aging, notions of manhood are similarly influenced by age, but crucially also shaped and constrained by wider biographical and social factors.

So how do men negotiate their way through age in terms of expressing and retaining the hegemonic ideal? Though there is an increasing literature relating masculinities and health, there is relatively little that addresses the experiences of men as they age. Indeed, literature on men's health remains dominated by epidemiological data and related research on risk. Such narratives serve to highlight male disadvantage as shown by mortality statistics and in risk factors such as being overweight, smoking and excessive alcohol consumption. Male lifestyles have become recognized as being dangerous to health and have prompted increasing reference to a contemporary 'crisis' afflicting men and masculinity. This overstated crisis, whilst referred in generic terms to men of all ages and stages, is seen to become more applicable to men as they become older and as masculine identity can no longer be portrayed or performed through a visually youthful male body. As Whitehead (2002: 200) states, 'masculinity is not static and unchanging – it changes and masculine identity which was once "inscribed" on the youthful male body becomes transformed just as the body is transformed through aging'. However, in the context of the destandardization or deinstitutionalization of the life course, many of the assumptions of body and age are radically disturbed.

The idea of the standardized life course has its origins in the emergence and bedding down of a classical modernity that was formed in the advanced industrial economies of Europe and North America in the first half of the twentieth century (Kohli 2007). The processes of industrialization and urbanization demanded that stable social structures were developed that organized the life courses of the vast majority of the population. These included education, work and retirement in addition to the domestic division of labour and the heterosexual male-headed household. As a result, a hegemonic masculinity could develop as an expression of these stable or as Bauman would call them 'solid' institutions (Bauman 2000). In part this reification of modernist social norms valorized a male embodiment that was both fit and functional for productive manual labour. Mandatory retirement represented a recognition that the productivity of older male labour was now a drag on productivity and it would be better if these men were taken out of the workforce so that labour efficiency could be maintained. Retired men therefore had to face the implication that they were both economically and socially redundant. Their masculinity was regarded as so vulnerable that in the UK women's state retirement ages were set at 60 instead of 65 so that wives would not potentially still be at work while their husbands were now drawing an old age pension.

However this was all to change. The classical modernist project started to fragment in the latter half of the twentieth century as both industrial labour and social norms started to be challenged by the advent of a more diverse economy and the rise of women's educational and employment opportunities. What Beck and his colleagues (2003) have called 'a revolution of side effects' saw, in the closing decades of the twentieth century, a profound transformation of social life where relative stability has been replaced by increased contingency in both employment and household relationships. The standardized life course was disrupted by repeated changes in working skills and organizations and the growth of 'precarious work' (Kalleberg 2009). In the domestic sphere assumptions about household forms and age-stratified activities such as motherhood have become much more varied, to the point that Beck (2007) has talked about the emergence of a new 'normativity of diversity'. In all of this the position of masculinity has been changed in two ways; first the need for a hegemonic masculinity becomes less as manual labour declines, and secondly the destandardization of the life course opens up opportunities for the Third Age to carve out a niche outside of employment and the labour process. Masculinity at older ages becomes more connected to a consumer lifestyle, as it does at earlier points in the lifespan, and is consequently as connected to narratives of fitness and vigour in later as it had been in earlier adult life. The one big difference is that retirement is no longer the cut-off point for maintaining a masculine identity; now it can continue as long as the individual can participate in Third Age cultures. Central to this change is consumer society and the way that it is oriented towards the body.

Consumer society, generation and the older body

Calasanti (2007: 358) argues that, as 'bodies serve as markers of age'; in Western culture consumer citizens are motivated to maintain the body in a perpetually youthful state. Indeed, according to some writers, 'western culture is predicated on the nexus of gendered youthfulness and consumption' (Schwaiger 2009: 275). As men enter into 'mid life' and encounter signs of bodily change and the beginnings of physical decline, masculine identity must then be expressed in other social and behaviour domains while still retaining an association with and remaining representative of the youthful, healthy ideal.

Calasanti (2007) draws attention to the role of the post-war 'baby boomer' generation in challenging the entrenched views and traditional notions and expectations of aging. As she sees it, this demographic cohort represents a cultural grouping who are seen to embody the postmodern ideal that individuals can control their bodies through lifestyle and consumer choices, where they can 'appear to age successfully and thus defend themselves against ageism' (Calasanti 2007: 359). This approach represents what could be represented as the mainstream approach to the intersecting issues of aging embodiment and masculinity in that it accepts that aging is a 'natural' process and that men along with women would accept it if it wasn't for the interventions of a youth orientated consumerism (Vincent 2006, 2009). Jones and Higgs (2010: 1514) on the other hand argue that the 'natural' life course has become destabilized along with traditional ideas of 'normal' and 'normative' aging and that 'the new reality of ageing intersects with the somatic aspects of consumer society based on difference and choice'. Rather than this being a form of 'false consciousness' or 'bad faith' on the part of the individual who does not want to grow old, it is part of a new reflexivity about aging, oriented towards the culture of fitness.

Zygmunt Bauman sees fitness not so much as a form of individual health but rather as a defining feature of a somaticized consumer culture in which the anxieties of a more contingent 'liquid modernity' are acted upon (Bauman 2000). Bauman argues that modern society has been transformed from a 'society of producers' to a 'society of consumers'. This is not just an economic transformation; it is also an ontological transformation whereby the body becomes the focus of individual action rather than being a factor of production, reproduction or military might. Bauman writes:

> The postmodern body is first and foremost a receiver of *sensations*, it imbibes and digests *experiences*; the capacity of being stimulated renders it an instrument of *pleasure*. That capacity is called fitness; obversely the 'state of unfitness' stands for languor, apathy, listlessness, dejection, a lackadaisical response to stimuli; for a shrinking or just 'below average' capacity for, and an interest in, new sensations and experiences.
> (Bauman 1995: 116)

The 'fitness' of the postmodern body is central to the practices of contemporary consumerism creating both discourses of 'rational' behaviour as well as leading to feelings of unease and dissatisfaction that in turn lead to further attempts at reaching contemporary ideals of fitness. In an important passage Bauman writes:

> 'Fitness' is to a consumer in the society of consumers what 'health' was to the society of producers. It is a certificate of 'being in', of belonging, of inclusion, of the right of residence. 'Fitness' knows no upper limit; it is, in fact, defined by the absence of limit ... However fit your body is – *you could make it fitter.* However fit it may be at the moment, there is always a vexing helping of 'unfitness' mixed in, coming to light or guessed at whenever you compare what you have experienced with the pleasures suggested by the rumours and sights of other people's joys which you have failed to experience thus far and can only imagine and dream of living through yourself. In the search for fitness, unlike in the case of health, there is no point at which you can say: now that I have reached it I may as well stop and hold onto and enjoy what I have. There is no 'norm' of fitness you can aim at and eventually attain.
> (Bauman 2005: 93)

In the light of this argument, it is not surprising that Jones and Higgs (2010) conclude that the culture of the Third Age leads to expectations that individuals will engage in all manner of anti-aging techniques in order to delay or at least slow down the progress of the marks of aging, and that this require a key role for the consumer market. This paradigm is further articulated through the ideas of 'healthy' aging where the reflexive self is expected to act agentically in pursuit of making the right choices for their future well-being (Rose 2001). These choices reflect the strong encouragement provided by a marketing discourse to individuals as 'consumers' to hide their physical signs of aging and to remain suspended in a state of 'agelessness'.

One outcome of these processes is the extension of mid-life into what previously would have been seen as old age. This is particularly pertinent given that those who contributed to the shaping of the post-war 'youth culture' – the baby boomers – are themselves either approaching retirement age or actually in it and so are happy to be seen as both redefining and confounding the meanings of aging. As Gilleard and Higgs (2011a) state, 'much of the physical reality of old age appears to have melted into the postmodern fiction of later life style', as changing experiences of leisure and consumerism challenge not just the narrative of aging but, as Basting (1998) points out, its performativity as well. This view echoes Featherstone's (1991) notion of the 'performing self', driven by consumption and by the moral imperative 'not to let one's self go' in an endless quest to enhance one's own health and marketability. Calasanti and Slevin (2001) posit this as a moral issue: individuals not only can but should exert control over their aging. All of this gives rise to attempts to separate a 'young' old, those aged between 55–74 who have expanding possibilities of not appearing or not performing as old, from those who are deemed the 'old' old, those aged 75 or older who have not. While rejecting a division based on age banding, Gilleard and Higgs (2011a) argue that it is within the lifestyles of the more recently retired that the cultural field of the Third Age is most fully emerging as the attitudes and experiences of the 1960s generation – born in a period of increasing economic affluence which privileged youth and youth culture – become the ones that are used to motivate the new circumstances of later life. The Third Age then is revealed in lifestyle rather than structured by status. Rather than be defined by a status as an ex-worker or seen in terms of social and cultural redundancy as in the category, old age pensioner, the lifestyle possibilities afforded by the Third Age offer the possibility of the construction of a lifestyle that allows for full participation in a consumer society . This generational habitus, to use a term Gilleard and Higgs (2011a) have adapted from Bourdieu, allows for the possibility of a lifestyle that is not so much about losing the attributes of youth as having a particular aversion to growing old, expressed by either denying or actively resisting aging or better still doing both (Gilleard and Higgs 2011a: 88). While, as in so many areas, access to this culture is dependent on the personal economic and social resources available, it is still the case that the emergence in later life of a generationally based form of consumption has changed the template for the whole of the field of aging and therefore of the discourses now possible for older people of both genders.

Masculinity, sexuality and growing older

As we have pointed out, as age and identity are negotiated across the life course, consumer discourses have targeted the body and have become central to anti-aging and age-resisting practices. Jones and Pugh (2005: 254–5, cited in Calasanti 2007) point out that: 'in a modern world in which the body is symbol of self expression ... not to resist signs of physical aging may be perceived as evidence of moral decline'. As new demands are made on the body, its appearance and its representation, the anti-aging industry and associated cosmetic practices not only promote the promise of maintaining youth, health and fitness, but crucially for our purposes also include maintaining an active sexual identity. Not only is sexuality part of the sensuous experiences central to Bauman's idea of a society of consumers but it is also something that is profoundly gendered as well as aged. Sexuality is valued as a fundamental dimension of 'being young' wherein individuals enact younger versions of femininity and masculinity in order to maintain a valued and embodied sexual identity for themselves (Katz and Marshall 2003). Conventionally, as previously noted, notions of masculinity are shaped around youthful images of male embodiment and as a consequence the aging male body is posited as facing potential 'demasculinisation' (Slevin 2010), given that the younger male body is held up as the ideal form of masculinity, perceived to be at the height of its productive capabilities. This productivity is seen to occur at a number of sites, economic, athletic and sexual, and as men age, their productivity within these sites decreases markedly (Slevin and Linneman 2010: 485). However if we accept the role of consumer lifestyle in helping spread the culture of the Third Age, it is also possible that consumer lifestyles might transcend the notion of idealized masculinity, operating at least at the level of the economic. The transformation of men from producers to consumers means that the primacy of economically productive masculinity may also have been transformed. The equation of labour productivity with hegemonic masculinity may only now persist in the realm of imagery rather than in terms of any real productivity. Consequently, if the retired man is no longer seen simply as a redundant or residual individual but instead as someone who is able to actively participate in the Third Age, then notions of being demasculinized may be short of the mark. In the world in which fitness is more important than health, a hegemonic masculinity may have been replaced by a series of potential realms of fitness; some of which older men can work towards and others which they may simply purchase.

The 'resexing' of aging bodies (Marshall and Katz 2006) might be one area where this is occurring. If conceptions of sexual normality and functionality are tied to masculine productivity, men in mid-life and beyond may choose to ensure their sexual fitness through the products provided by the pharmaceutical industry. With references to the development of 'masculinity in a pill', Loe (2006) claims that in the 'Viagra era' the male body is re-emerging as a site for confidence and control:

> With Viagra a highly successful masculine empowerment campaign is underway ... which promises to produce and enhance male bodies, confidence levels and overall spirits ... The little blue pill is envisioned as cutting edge biotechnology and used as a cultural and material tool in the production and achievement of 'true' manhood.
>
> (Loe 2006: 43)

Whilst some like Calasanti and King (2007) see this as not just extending a sexualized identity for men but also as a way of maintaining a previous position of power, not all commentators are so critical. Hockey and James (2003) argue that this extension of a sexualized identity should be a cause for celebration rather than concern and add that the persistence of a sexualized identity into later life among men has been endorsed by Viagra as 'an ageing male population wish to recapture youthful potency via a chemical remedy' (Hockey and James 2003: 151). Returning to our earlier point, while drugs like Viagra and Cialis may seem to restore an earlier potency to men and therefore operate in terms of a simple discourse of masculinity, it is probably more important to note that it also illustrates the point that there are different routes to 'fitness' in later life. Whether this fitness is desired by all members of the older population is another question, but the fact that 'age' can be reversed does underpin the increasing diversity of later life experiences such that what is normal or indeed normative is much more difficult to ascertain.

Another dimension of this transformation of the relationship between masculinity and aging is the recognition of the male menopause (or andropause) as a medical condition (Carruthers 1996) with testosterone replacement therapy being increasingly offered as a supplement to 'treat' the symptoms of aging. There is a long history of interest in the role of testosterone and its role in situating masculinity (see Watkins' chapter in this volume; Roberts 2007), including its identification with decreased sex drive, sexual dysfunction as well as a decrease in competitiveness. Testosterone is portrayed by some as a 'miraculous substance, with amazing power to restore or enhance masculinity' (Szymczak and Conrad 2006). Others such as Watkins takes a more sanguine view, showing that the emergence of this therapy has not been unproblematic nor without risks. However as Roberts (2007: 129) points out, the 'problems' of the aging male provide an 'appealing new market for pharmaceutical and biomedical products' which not only lead to new forms of medicalization but also, through their links to cosmetic surgery and anti-impotence medication, contribute to new arenas of consumption.

In offering solutions to the 'crisis of masculinity' brought about in part by aging we can once again see the importance of anti-aging medicines and techniques in the construction of older men's lives and identities. The boundary between what is anti-aging technique and what is purported to be a medical procedure is becoming as blurred among men as it already is among women. For men, signs of aging – related to sexual performance and physicality – are increasingly becoming medicalized and the aging process pathologized. In terms of a malleable physical identity anti-aging practices are more obviously evident for the postponement of aging for middle-aged women – surgical techniques such as breast reshaping, liposuction or face lifts help obliterate or disguise the changes bought by age (Hockey and James 2003). Offering to preserve or restore youthful performance, pharmacological intervention therefore provides men the opportunity to retain a sexualized masculine identity, at a time when the body itself can no longer be identified with the 'hegemonic' fit, active and youthful masculine body. While, according to Hartley (2003), the medicalization of male sexual 'fitness' is an interesting and rare case of men's sexual problems having been medicalized before women's, this may be because it very obviously fits in with the valorization of youthfulness that is an intrinsic part of Third Age culture and at a single stroke removes one of the main lines of fracture between older and younger men insofar as it relates to their capacity to act as 'sensation seekers' in a consumer society. The example of Viagra helping to eradicate impotence – the 'scourge of many old men's bodies' – not only reflects moves to 'medicalize underperformance' (Conrad and Potter 2000) but also altered expectations of aging.

Returning to the idea of fitness in the culture of the Third Age we can see that instead of a 'healthy' male being characterized by optimum physical functioning, older men whose bodily functioning may become limited choose to adopt other options. Visser *et al.* (2009) suggest that men may be able to create a viable masculine identity by using competence in one masculine domain to compensate for lack of competence in other masculine domains. We have seen this in relation to pharmacological interventions such as Viagra which not only restores but improves competence in the domain of sexual function and performance. As contemporary expectations about health, fitness and sexuality have pushed men to maintain youthful performance in all aspects of their lives (Luciano 2001: 203, cited in Rosenfeld and Faircloth 2006), the process of medicalization enables men to retain some of the essentially 'masculine' and embodied qualities of youth. It becomes one of a number of strategies that have to be adopted in the much more contingent world of 'liquid modernity'. Those participating in the cultures of the Third Age have to be adept at negotiating the different discourses of aging with agency. For men the collapse of the 'society of producers' has opened up opportunities that were largely absent when their status (or non-status) as a producer determined their fate. However, this does not mean that aging and aging bodies are any more acceptable because they are male than they were in the past. The key factor is whether or not the older man can maintain a form of 'ageless' masculinity from the resources available and still show that he is capable of engaging in a culture of fitness and of choice.

The negotiation of the Third and Fourth Ages

Gilleard and Higgs (2011a) argue that one of the central features of the culture of the Third Age is resistance to being ascribed with the status of old age. By actively excluding 'old age' and 'agedness' and by distancing the Third Age from the signs of bodily aging, those participating in this generational field have chosen cultural agency over biological structure. As this chapter has argued, this fits in with the emergent discourse of reflexivity and fitness in later life, however it does draw a sharp distinction from those who are defined by the infirmities and dependencies of old age. Engagement with the culture of the Third Age demands an active working on maintaining youthfulness and for men a capacity to enact dimensions of masculinity. However, in spite of all the effort there still exists the possibility that one day prevention will not be possible. The pressures of maintaining 'performing fit, healthy, sexualised' lifestyles has pushed agedness to a horizon, a point where the capacities of the sick body can no longer signify youthfulness and full participation in meaningful consumption will no longer be possible (Tulle-Winton 1999). This position – described as the Fourth Age – represents the physical dependency and mental confusion associated with conventional accounts of old age, where the 'frail' are at the limits of their functional capacity (Gilleard and Higgs 2010, 2011b).

The images associated with the Fourth Age are those which traditionally signify 'old' age – grey hair, wrinkled skin. The very length of one's life is measured against a presumed loss of functional capacities. Gilleard and

Higgs (2011b) propose that mapping old age as a Fourth Age imaginary serves two purposes – first to help distance longer lives and later lifestyles from what they term the 'abjection of old age', whilst intensifying 'the horror with which real old age is viewed, a horror at the otherness of the orphaned and decaying body' (ibid. 138). Fittingly this illustrates how the imaging of 'older' people – and therefore older men – is encumbered with negativity from the outset.

> The dominant discourses of youth and middle age combine to further 'white out' the presences of older men. These pre-death older men who have already lost out in the 'aging stakes' are stereotyped as genderless, even emasculated, such that the social construction of older men maintains that old men are not men at all.
> (Thompson 1994: 18)

Hearn (1995: 101) adds that older men in contemporary society are, 'relatively redundant, even invisible ... in terms of life itself'.

The power of the Fourth Age, argue Gilleard and Higgs (2010, 2011b), lies not in its 'lived experience' (something that they argue is more or less incapable of direct subjective accounting) but in its capacity to act as a 'social imaginary', a collective mental representation which because it represents extreme levels of physical dependency and mental decline acts as a metaphorical 'black hole' from which nothing can escape. The circumstances represented by the Fourth Age pose a threat to those seen to be on its boundary. The lack of agency, independence and physical control, which are all components of this categorical imaginary, can all too easily be transferred to those attempting to maintain their roles as participants in the Third Age. Problems of mobility may indicate subclinical risks; falls may be precursors to diagnoses of frailty; and forgetfulness may be early warning signs of mental confusion.

It is not surprising that, given the symbolic role of the Fourth Age, a whole platform of preventative techniques and treatments both medical and non-medical has emerged to promote fitness or retard decline. These particularly focus on mental functioning, with commercial products for 'brain training' becoming available as well as pharmaceutical compounds being developed for the treatment of Mild Cognitive Impairment (MCI), a condition identified as a 'pre-dementia' (Williams *et al.* 2012). What these interventions share with the more conventional health promotion techniques and products is the articulation of a desire still to be able to make a claim to be agentic, to be a participant in the Third Age and not be ascribed the status of existing in the Fourth Age where, as we have seen, women and particularly men become invisible. Within these sets of circumstances the capacity to perform any sort of masculinity is almost impossible and unlike the transgressive forms of abjection proposed by some authors, represents an abjection that cannot give rise to any positive possibilities.

Conclusion

This chapter has been concerned with trying to situate masculinity within the changing nature of later life. It has used the prism of the Third and Fourth Ages to think through how conventional approaches to embodied masculinity that have privileged younger and working age men have been challenged both by the social changes to employment and retirement that have created a more diverse environment for the expression of later life lifestyles, and by the anti-aging interventions provided by biomedicine and the market. The chapter concurs with Minichiello *et al.*'s (2000) point that old age is a time when self-identity is challenged and that people tend to avoid identifying themselves as old in order to avoid the exclusion that such statuses bring about. The Third Age is based upon such a position to the extent that it rejects entirely any connection with a putative Fourth Age. In this cultural environment masculinity can be reconstructed as an engagement with any number of anti-aging discourses, including conventional health promotion, bodywork and pharmaceutical interventions. The concept 'forever functional' can act as a response to the more demanding if more unattainable tropes of hegemonic masculinity, by providing another route to a 'fitness' that is desired. Like all panaceas, however, the desire to maintain an 'ageless self' is ultimately confronted with some of the limitations of the human body and, while negotiation of the boundaries between the Third and Fourth Ages will occur, the impact of being sucked into the Fourth Age removes any possibility of agency let alone masculinity. The difficulty with previous renderings of the impact of old age on masculinity is that they have not understood that this location is not representative of contemporary later life as a whole and have therefore subsumed all of post-working life under the same banner of frailty and dependency. In short, we would therefore argue that an understanding of the significance of the Third and Fourth Ages is essential if the contemporary nature of masculinity and its relationship to aspirational medicine is to be fully explored.

References

Basting, A. D. (1998) *The Stages of Age: Performing Age in Contemporary American Culture*, Ann Arbor, MI: University of Michigan Press.
Bauman, Z. (1995) *Life in Fragments: Essays in Postmodern Morality*, Oxford: Blackwell.
Bauman, Z. (2000) *Liquid Modernity*, Cambridge: Polity.
Bauman, Z. (2005) *Liquid Life*, Cambridge: Polity.
Beck, U. (2007) 'Beyond class and nation: Reframing social inequalities in a globalizing world', *British Journal of Sociology*, 58(4): 679–705.
Beck, U., Bonss, W., and Lau, C. (2003) 'The theory of reflexive modernisation, problematic, hypotheses and research programme', *Theory, Culture and Society*, 20(2): 1–33.
Calasanti, T. (2007) 'Bodacious berry, potency wood and the aging monster: Gender and age relations in anti-aging ads', *Social Forces*, 86(1): 335–55.

Calasanti, T., and King, N. (2007) '"Beware of the estrogen assault": Ideals of old manhood in anti-aging advertisements', *Journal of Aging Studies*, 21: 357–68.
Calasanti, T., and Slevin, K. (2001) *Gender, Social Inequalities and Aging*. Walnut Creek, CA: Alta Maria Press.
Carruthers, M. (1996) *Male Menopause: Restoring Vitality and Virility*, New York: HarperCollins.
Coles, T. (2009) 'Negotiating the field of masculinity: The production and reproduction of multiple dominant masculinities', *Men and Masculinities*, 12(1): 30–44.
Conrad, P., and Potter, D. (2000) 'From hyperactive children to ADHD adults: Observations on the expansion of medical categories', *Social Problems* 47: 559–82.
Faircloth, C. A. (2003) *Aging Bodies: Images and Everyday Experience*, Walnut Creek, CA: AltaMira Press.
Featherstone, M. (1991) 'The body in consumer culture', in M. Featherstone, M. Hepworth and B.S. Turner (eds), *The Body: Social Process and Cultural Theory*, London: Sage.
Gilleard C and Higgs P. (2000) *Cultures of Ageing: Self, Citizen and the Body*, Harlow: Prentice Hall.
Gilleard, C., and Higgs, P. (2005) *Contexts of Ageing: Class, Cohort and Community*, Cambridge: Polity Press.
Gilleard, C., and Higgs, P. (2010) 'Theorizing the fourth age: Aging without agency', *Aging and Mental Health*, 14: 121–8.
Gilleard, C., and Higgs, P. (2011a) 'The Third Age as a cultural field', in D. Carr and K. Komp (eds), *Gerontology in the Era of the Third Age* (pp. 33–50), New York: Springer.
Gilleard, C., and Higgs, P. (2011b) 'Ageing abjection and embodiment in the Fourth Age', *Journal of Aging Studies*, 25: 135–42.
Grenier, A. (2007) 'Constructions of frailty in the English language, care practice and the lived experience', *Ageing and Society*, 27: 425–45.
Hartley, H. (2003) '"Big Pharma" in our bedrooms: An analysis of the medicalization of women's sexual problems', in M. S. Segal and V. Demos (eds), *Gender Perspectives on Health and Medicine: Key Themes, Advances in Gender Research*, 7 (pp. 1–9), Oxford: Elsevier Press.
Hearn, J. (1995) 'Imaging the aging of men', in M. Featherstone and A. Wernick (eds), *Images of Aging: Cultural Representations of Later Life* (pp. 97–117). London: Routledge.
Higgs, P., and Jones, I. R. (2009) *Medical Sociology and Old Age: Towards a Sociology of Health in Later Life*, London: Routledge.
Hockey, J., and James, A. (2003) *Social Identities across the Life Course*, New York: Palgrave Macmillan.
Jones, I. R., and Higgs, P. (2010) 'The natural, the normal and the normative: Contested terrains in ageing and old age', *Social Science and Medicine*, 71: 1513–19.
Jones, J., and Pugh, S. (2005) 'Ageing gay men: Lessons from the sociology of embodiment', *Men and Masculinities*, 7(3): 248–60.
Kalleberg, A. L. (2009) 'Precarious work, insecure workers: Employment relations in transition', *American Sociological Review*, 74(1): 1–22.
Katz, S., and Marshall, B. L. (2003) 'New sex for old: Lifestyle, consumerism, and the ethics of aging well', *Journal of Aging Studies*, 17(1): 3–16.

Kohli, M. (2007) 'The institutionalization of the life course: Looking back to look ahead', *Research in Human Development*, 4(3–4): 253–71.
Leontowitsch, M., Higgs, P., Stevenson, F., and Jones, I. R. (2010) 'Taking care of yourself in later life: A qualitative study into the use of non-prescription medicines by people aged 60+', *Health*, 14: 213–31.
Loe, M. (2006) 'The Viagra blues: Embracing or resisting the Viagra body', in D. Rosenfeld and C. A. Faircloth (eds), *Medicalized Masculinities*, Philadelphia, PA: Temple University Press.
Lucianno, L. (2001) *Looking Good: Male Body Image in Modern America*, New York: Hill & Wang.
Marshall, B. L., and Katz, S. (2006) 'From Androgyny to Androgens: Re-sexing the Aging Body', in T. Calasanti and K. Slevin (eds), *Age Matters* (pp. 75–98), New York: Routledge.
Minichiello, V., Browne, J., and Kendig, H. (2000) 'Perceptions and consequences of ageism: views of older people', *Ageing and Society*, 20(3): 253–78.
Roberts, C. (2007) *Messengers of Sex: Hormones, Biomedicine and Feminism*, Cambridge, Cambridge University Press.
Rose, N. (2001) 'The politics of life itself', *Theory, Culture and Society*, 18(6): 1–30.
Rosenfeld, D., and Faircloth, C. A. (eds) (2006), *Medicalized Masculinities*, Philadelphia, PA: Temple University Press.
Russell, C. (2007) 'What do older women and men want? Gender differences in the "lived experience" of ageing', *Current Sociology*, 55(2): 173–92.
Schwaiger, E. (2009) 'Performing youth: Ageing, ambiguity and bodily integrity', *Social Identities*, 15(2): 273–84.
Slevin, K. F. (2010) '"If I had lots of money ... I'd have a body makeover:" managing the aging body', *Social Forces*, 88 (3): 1003–1020.
Slevin, K. F., and Linneman, T. J. (2010) 'Old gay men's bodies and masculinities', *Men and Masculinities*, 12(4): 483–507.
Szymczak, J. E., and Conrad, P. (2006) 'Medicalizing the aging male body: Andropause and baldness', in D. Rosenfeld and C.A. Faircloth (eds), *Medicalized Masculinities* (pp. 89–111), Philadelphia, PA: Temple University Press.
Thompson, E. H. (1994) 'Older men as invisible men in contemporary society', in E. H. Thompson (ed), *Older Men's Lives* (pp. 1–21), Thousand Oaks, CA: Sage.
Tulle-Winton, E. (1999) 'Growing old and resistance: Towards a new cultural economy of old age?', *Ageing and Society*, 19: 281–99.
Vincent, J. (2006) 'Ageing contested: Anti-ageing science and the cultural construction of old age', *Sociology*, 40(4): 681–98.
Vincent, J. (2009) 'Ageing, anti-ageing and anti-anti-ageing: Who are the progressives in the debate on human biological ageing?', *Medicine Studies*, 1: 197–208.
Visser, R. O., Smith, J., and McDonnell, E. J. (2009) '"That's not masculine": Masculine capital and health-related behaviour', *Journal of Health Psychology*, 14(7): 1047–58.
Watson, J. (2000) *Male Bodies: Health, Culture and Identity*, Buckingham: Open University Press.
Whitehead, S. M. (2002) *Men and Masculinities*, Cambridge: Polity Press.
Williams, S., Higgs, P., and Katz, S. (2012) 'Neuroculture, active ageing and the "older brain": problems, promises and prospects', *Sociology of Health & Illness*, 34(1): 64–78.

2 Testosterone and the pharmaceuticalization of male aging

Elizabeth Siegel Watkins

Americans who watched the 2010 World Series on television also saw many commercials, one of which advertised awareness of a medical condition plaguing men of a certain age. 'Millions of men 45 and older just don't feel like they used to,' the narrator intoned. After describing the symptoms – low energy, low sex drive and moodiness – he went on to inform viewers, 'It could be a treatable condition called low testosterone or low T.' 'Don't blame it on aging,' he advised, urging sufferers instead to 'Talk to your doctor, and go to IsItLowT.com to find out more.' Those who followed his directions to the website found a 'Low T Quiz,' which identified seven additional symptoms, making a total of ten: body changes, sexual dysfunction, decreased strength and/or endurance, loss of height, deterioration in ability to play sports, deterioration in work performance and falling asleep after dinner. The site recommended that men who had acknowledged even just a few of the signs print out the completed quiz, take it to their doctors and ask if they should be tested for low testosterone.

This television commercial and its companion website were sponsored by Abbott Laboratories, which had recently acquired the Belgian-based Solvay Pharmaceuticals for $6.6 billion. Solvay manufactured AndroGel, a topical ointment that dominated the testosterone market, accounting for more than 70 percent of all testosterone prescriptions. The 'Is It Low T' advertisement made four points, three explicit and one implicit. First, it clearly separated the condition of low testosterone from normal aging. Second, it convinced men that the proper course of action was to seek medical help. Third, it suggested that the condition could be diagnosed with a quantitative measurement of testosterone levels. Anyone who had seen a drug commercial in the past decade could intuit the fourth, unstated, point: the promise of a pharmaceutical solution to this medical problem.

The use of the male sex hormone, testosterone, to treat this constellation of symptoms was nothing new. Soon after testosterone was discovered, isolated and synthesized in the laboratory in 1935, drug companies began to produce testosterone products for physicians to give to their middle-aged male patients who complained of fatigue, irritability, low libido and impotence. From the late 1930s to the mid-1950s, many doctors in the United States and Europe prescribed a regimen of intramuscular injections of testosterone to counter the effects of what was then called the male climacteric. Throughout this period, conflicting evidence and opinions appeared in medical journals about the treatment, diagnosis and even the very existence of the male climacteric. Some authors argued that it was a real physical condition, caused by a deficiency of the male sex hormone and alleviated by hormone replacement therapy. Others rejected this endocrinological aetiology, arguing instead that the symptoms resulted from a psychoneurotic condition, brought on by the social stresses and economic pressures of modern life. While the former group drew parallels between the female menopause and the male climacteric, the latter objected to the emasculating notion that men could suffer from anything like a women's condition (Watkins 2008).

By the late 1950s, the psychological explanation had won the debate. The syndrome was reframed as the somatic expression of stress-induced psychic woes, and patients were prescribed tranquillizers instead of hormones. Although journalists and medical popularizers writing in the popular press continued to promote the notion that aging men, like their female counterparts, could suffer from debilitating symptoms caused by decreasing hormone levels, clinicians and medical researchers ignored the topic. Discussion of the male climacteric and testosterone replacement therapy virtually disappeared from the medical literature in North America, Europe, and Australia for the next forty years[1] (Watkins 2007b).

Then, in the late 1990s, articles on male menopause began to reappear in medical journals. The fusty term 'climacteric' was replaced by the more modern-sounding 'andropause', and once again physicians debated whether or not men experienced androgen deficiency that was in any way comparable to the oestrogen deficiency of menopause. The subject gained momentum, and in the decade from 2000 to 2009, there were ten times as many medical journal articles on andropause as compared to the previous decade of 1990–9 and fifty times as many as compared to the 1980s. Why, after four decades of neglect by the medical profession, did a new generation of doctors take up the study, diagnosis and treatment of male menopause? How and why did medicine reframe the concept of male menopause – from climacteric to andropause to androgen deficiency in the aging male (ADAM) to late-onset hypogonadism to low T – in the late 1990s and 2000s? This chapter addresses these questions, locating the answers in two evolving trends: first, a changing conception of masculinity, particularly with respect to health and aging, and second, a reductionism in medicine that based the diagnosis of disease on quantitative measures.

Masculinity in crisis in the 1990s: boys and behaviour, men and medicine

The origins of the revival of interest in the possibility of male menopause within the medical profession are rooted in the cultural context and medical fashion of the early 1990s. A prominent cultural figure at that time was Robert Bly, the poet-turned-men's movement leader, who believed that ever since the Industrial Revolution had driven men out to the workplace, their absence from the home had left boys with no suitable mentors to shepherd them from boyhood to manhood. Bly wrote a bestseller in 1990, *Iron John: A Book about Men*, which used the allegory of a Grimm Brothers' fairy tale to help men discover the pathway to maturity. He and others of the movement's leaders also held men-only self-help workshops, which received ample coverage by the popular press. As Richard Stengel, writing in *Time* magazine, put it: 'The men's movement is a misnomer. It is neither political like the civil rights movement nor activist like the women's movement. It is a convenient catchphrase for something that is bubbling up around the country – men attending consciousness-raising seminars, men tramping off for weekends in the woods, men crying, men laughing, men drumming – which suggest that the state of American guyness is kind of shaky' (Stengel 1991). To many contemporaries, this movement seemed to be evidence of a sort of crisis in masculinity.

In the realm of health care, a number of studies found that men were more likely than women to engage in risky behaviour, less likely to engage in health-promoting behaviour, less likely to visit the doctor and more likely to die from all of the leading causes of death. Sociologists attributed these discrepancies to men's determination to appear tough and macho; the performance of masculinity, they hypothesized, prevented men from taking care of their health (Courtenay 2000). A 1991 survey of men aged 50 and over, for example, found that almost half of those who admitted to being depressed had not discussed it with anyone (Courtenay 2000). By contrast, older women seemed more and more comfortable talking about their bodies and their health. In the early 1990s, menopause went public, as magazines and newspapers wrote about aging baby boomer women.

These women, unlike their male counterparts, did visit their doctors, and many of them came away with prescriptions for oestrogen. By 1992, the Premarin brand of oestrogen replacement therapy became the most widely prescribed drug in America. In 1992, the American College of Physicians recommended that 'all women, regardless of race, should consider preventive hormone therapy' after menopause 'to prevent disease and to prolong life' (Watkins 2007a: 240). Numerous observational studies suggested that women who took oestrogen had a decreased risk of developing osteoporosis and cardiovascular disease, and women who took oestrogen reported anecdotally that they looked and felt better than their non-oestrogenated selves.

With positive reports of the benefits of oestrogen for post-menopausal women filling the pages of both medical journals and popular periodicals, some physicians began to wonder if aging men might also benefit from hormone replacement.[2] Medical journal articles in the 1980s and early 1990s had reported that testosterone levels decreased steadily in older men, but the effects of this decline were unknown. A 1991 meta-analysis of the association between testosterone and male aging published in the *Journal of Clinical Epidemiology* observed that 'the study of testosterone is likely to be prominent in future epidemiological work on endocrine function and the clinical treatment of age-related diseases' (Gray *et al.* 1991: 671).

Andropause and testosterone began to creep back into the medical literature in the mid-1990s. In 1995, an article in *Geriatrics* posed the question: 'Hormone Replacement Therapy for Men: Has the Time Come?' (Weksler 1995). In 1998, an article on male hormone replacement therapy and andropause in *Endocrinology and Metabolism Clinics* began with an explicit proposal to redress the imbalance in attention to male and female aging:

> Although hormone replacement therapy (HRT) for postmenopausal women has been studied, discussed, and practiced for years, there has been much less focus on hypogonadal disorders of the adult male and male HRT. This is manifested both in clinical practice, where the symptoms of adult hypogonadism in the male are often attributed to other problems, denied by the patient, and underrecognized by the physician, and in research, which has produced few data on the long-term risks and benefits of androgen replacement therapy in middle age and beyond. The use of testosterone therapy to prevent or reverse aspects of male 'andropause' is a topic of growing interest.
>
> (Tenover 1998: 970)

The notion that older men were being given short shrift by medical researchers and practitioners was also expressed in an article published in *Annals of Long Term Care*, titled 'Equal Time for the Older Male: Pathophysiology, Evaluation, and Management of Male Osteoporosis'. Osteoporosis affected more women than men, so it had been considered primarily a disease of post-menopausal females. The author contended that this labelling had resulted in female-focused research that 'neglect(ed) the threat the disease poses to elderly men'. He also charged the medical profession with clinical neglect, as women were encouraged to have their bone density measured, but no such recommendations were made for men (Orwoll 2001).

One of the strongest and most vocal supporters of the legitimacy of male menopause and its treatment with testosterone replacement was the British physician Malcolm Carruthers, who set up the Centre for Men's Health in Harley Street in 1988. In 1996, HarperCollins published his book, *Male Menopause: Restoring Vitality and Virility*, intended for a popular audience (Carruthers 1996). Carruthers scolded both men and their (male) physicians for allowing 'their macho self-image' to impede their recognition of the male version of menopause, in a mocking account of the typical doctor–patient encounter:

When, after ignoring or denying his condition for months or even years, the quietly desperate man goes to see a doctor, all he is told is: 'So you feel tired, dispirited, exhausted and your sex life is non-existent? So your wife had the same symptoms when she went through the menopause and got hormones from her gynaecologist which revitalized her so much you can't keep up? That doesn't apply to *you* – there's no such thing as the male menopause or male hormone replacement therapy. Just forget it and take these anti-depressants – they'll make us both feel better'.
(Carruthers 1996: p. ix)

Carruthers rejected the common medical wisdom of the past forty years – that men did not experience an andropause and that their symptoms should be treated with psychopharmaceuticals – and endeavoured to 're-establish the concept (of male menopause) and the benefits of treatment (with testosterone) once and for all' (Carruthers 1996: p. xvi).

Technology and testosterone: the patch

By the time Carruthers wrote his male menopause manifesto, a new delivery system for testosterone had come onto the market. Prior to this technological development, physicians who wanted to prescribe testosterone had three options. The most common form was by injection; oral tablets and pellet implants were also available but were used much less frequently. Oral tablets, which at first glance would seem to be the preferable form, had earned a tainted reputation because they had dangerous physiological side effects and also because they were used primarily by athletes looking to bulk up their muscles. A testosterone skin cream was available in France, but it had the problem of rubbing off on men's female partners, causing virilization.

The new delivery system was a transdermal patch. When applied to the skin, the patch released a continuous dose of the drug, keeping its concentration in the blood relatively consistent. This method offered a clear advantage over the injection, which produced an initial rapid elevation of testosterone in the blood that then slowly ebbed away. In October 1993, Testoderm won FDA approval for the treatment of hypogonadism in men (FDA 1993).

Testoderm was produced by the Alza Corporation, which had developed most of the other existing transdermal products (Alza 1996). Alza submitted its New Drug Application (NDA) for Testoderm to the FDA in the summer of 1987, well before articles on male menopause had become prevalent in the medical literature. The indications for use of the approved product made no mention of aging or andropause; the package label (for physicians and pharmacists) listed only primary hypogonadism (failure of the testes due to a variety of causes) and hypogonadotrophic hypogonadism (causes by problems in the pituitary or hypothalamus of the brain) as indications for use in adults (the product had not been evaluated in males under the age of 18) (FDA 1993).

Testoderm had one key feature that prevented its widespread acceptance among men being treated for hypogonadism: it had to be applied daily to the skin of the scrotum. Another company, Theratech, predicted that a patch that could be worn anywhere else on the body would be more successful; it submitted an NDA for its version of a testosterone skin patch in 1994 and won FDA approval to market Androderm one year later. The Androderm system consisted of two patches to be applied every evening to the back, abdomen, thigh or upper arm, in rotation to avoid skin irritation at any one site (FDA 1995). Alza responded quickly with its own non-scrotal patch; Testoderm-TTS was approved in 1997. By this time, FDA regulators recognized that the market for testosterone might be expanded beyond the group of patients with congenital or acquired hypogonadism. Jean L. Fourcroy, the FDA medical officer responsible for the medical review of Testoderm-TTS prior to its approval, noted: 'There are a large number of men requiring testosterone replacement. The current estimates are increasing with the growing realization that the aging male population may also need hormone replacement therapy (HRT). *Androgen delivery systems are therefore a booming business*' (FDA 1997: A11; emphasis added)

In 1999, American physicians wrote a total of 648,000 prescriptions for testosterone (Liverman and Blazer 2004: 24). Data on the proportion of testosterone that was sold as transdermal patches for that year are not available, but by 2000, Androderm had captured 30 percent of the retail market, and the two versions of Testoderm together accounted for another 27 percent (Mehta 2009). Overall, the annual number of testosterone prescriptions was growing at a rapid rate; the figure in 1999 was more than five times that of 1992. However, testosterone use paled in comparison to oestrogen use. In 1999, 89.6 million oestrogen prescriptions were filled. In other words, for every 138 women on oestrogen, just one man was taking testosterone.

The game changer: Viagra

And then came Viagra. The little blue pill that would revolutionize older men's health care, carrying testosterone along in its wake, was approved by the FDA in March 1998 for the treatment of erectile dysfunction, formerly known as impotence. Viagra made erectile dysfunction, specifically, and men's health issues, more generally, acceptable to talk about and to seek treatment for. Pfizer, the maker of Viagra, began to advertise Viagra on television in early 1999 and rolled out new ad campaigns on a regular basis. The product was phenomenally successful, reaching blockbuster status more quickly than any other drug in history (Loe 2004).

What Viagra did for impotent men was to remove their inability to achieve an erection from the realm of the psyche and to recast it as a purely physiological malfunction. Men did not need psychotherapy, Viagra proved; all they needed was a little chemical assistance in the corpus cavernosal tissue of their penises. As sociologist Jennifer Fishman has demonstrated, Viagra represented the end point of a medical transition that began in the 1980s to 'organicize' impotence, 'relocating (it) from a problem of the mind to a problem of the body' (Fishman 2007: 246). This is precisely what andropause advocates aspired to do: relocate the source of men's mid-life symptoms from the mind to the body, specifically to the decreased production of testosterone by the testes.

Attention to the health issues of older men got a further boost in 1998 with the inaugural issue of a journal called *The Aging Male*, published by the newly formed International Society for the Study of the Aging Male (ISSAM). In the first editorial, Bruno Lunenfeld, an endocrinologist from Bar-Ilan University in Israel, charged the medical, behavioural and social sciences with 'oversight, absence of focusing, disconnection and, most of all, lack of interdisciplinary collaboration' on the subject of male aging (Lunenfeld 1998: 1). He called for more research, specifically into hormone replacement therapy, which could improve men's health by 'preventing the preventable and delaying the inevitable'. He continued with a comparison between the sexes: 'Evidence is available that such interventions reduce cardiovascular disease and osteoporosis and may delay the onset of Alzheimer's disease in women. There is an urgent need to obtain such information in men' (Lunenfeld 1998: 6).

ISSAM held its first general meeting in Geneva in February 1998. The composition of this organization was truly international, with delegates from all over the developed world. The forty-three members of the Scientific Advisory Board represented twenty-four countries on five continents, indicating that male aging was a transnational health concern. ISSAM published its mission statement in a 1999 issue of *The Aging Male*. The rationale for the existence of the Society was introduced in terms of a comparison between men and women:

> In the last two decades, research has concentrated on the effects of the menopause in aging women and hormone replacement therapy for women now has proven benefits. A number of organizations exist whose aim is to improve the quality of life of the aging woman. Studies on the aging process in males have been neglected ... The aging of the human male requires special consideration.
>
> (ISSAM 1999: 6)

The organization intended to redress this imbalance by establishing a 'global forum' to promote, support and disseminate scientific, medical, psychosocial and socioeconomic research and clinical applications to improve the lives of aging men.

Thus, by the end of the 1990s, aging men had captured the attention of medical and popular culture. With the establishment of an international scientific society dedicated to the study of older men and the media buzz about Viagra and erectile dysfunction, clinicians could bring andropause out of the closet. The context for this development had been set: changing notions of masculinity and men's roles, as discussed above, had brought about a re-evaluation of men's health needs. Recall Carruthers's scorn for men's 'macho self-image', which represented this larger shift in conceptions and performances of masculinity in relation to health and aging. As more and more women turned to oestrogen to maintain their femininity and to prevent age-related diseases, men also turned to medicine to avoid the de-masculinizing effects of aging. There is a sort of paradox inherent in men performing in a less traditionally masculine way (i.e. seeking medical and pharmaceutical help) in order to regain the masculinity associated with youthfulness.

Sociologist Barbara Marshall has argued that the renewed interest in the diagnosis and treatment of male menopause resulted from a revised cultural narrative of aging and sexuality that constructed the aging male body as a site for biomedical intervention. Certainly the Viagra story supports this contention. Marshall further explains that, in this new narrative, aging was equated with de-masculinization, and in order for men to be fully masculine, they had to be fully sexual. Testosterone therapy built on Viagra's promise to keep men sexually functional, and therefore still masculine (Marshall 2007). I suggest that Marshall's thesis can be expanded by including other markers of manliness and youthfulness, besides sexual function, in the analysis. That is, muscle strength, fitness and endurance were also critical to the diagnosis of andropause, a condition that would ultimately require medical, and pharmaceutical, attention. Viagra could be prescribed to treat erectile dysfunction, but it did not address the other symptoms of mid-life malaise: low libido, fatigue, irritability and so on. Hormone replacement therapy, however, could fulfil this function, if these symptoms could be positively linked to testosterone deficiency. This leads us to the second trend that facilitated the legitimization of testosterone therapy for older men: reductionism in medicine. While Marshall has ably described the broader cultural changes that enabled the renaissance of male menopause, I focus here on the medical-industrial complex, that is, on the mutually reinforcing developments in the science and practice of clinical medicine and the commercial designs of the pharmaceutical enterprise that produced the diagnosis and treatment of what came to be 'a treatable condition called Low T'.

From andropause to 'Low T'

In the early 2000s, a robust discourse on andropause appeared in the medical literature, mostly in specialist journals. Each of these articles began with a commentary on the semantic problem of what to call the set of symptoms that seemed to be related to declining testosterone levels in aging men. One representative article described the inadequacy of all the terms in use. It rejected male menopause because there was, obviously, no cessation of menstruation in men; viropause, because there was no loss of virilization;

and male climacteric, because that term did not relate the syndrome to androgen levels. ADAM, the article noted, was sometimes morphed into PADAM (partial androgen deficiency in the aging male) or AAAD (aging-associated androgen deficiency). Reluctantly, the author chose to use andropause, 'because it is the only term that relates the syndrome of age-related pathological changes with the gradual and progressive decline in T levels'. Furthermore, he noted, 'Andropause is a term also used commonly by experts in the field and by lay persons *because it retains some analogy to menopause in women*' (Matsumoto 2002: M76; emphasis added).

This inaccurate analogy between men and women bothered clinicians and researchers. 'Owing to the similarity between most of the symptoms in men and women the term "menopause" gained popularity and has unfortunately stuck,' lamented two British physicians from the WellMan Clinic in London (Gould and Petty 2000: 858). Consistent coverage of the male menopause in newspapers and magazines had conditioned the public to accept that term, however incorrectly it described the male condition. The problem was that the symptoms of menopause and andropause were almost exactly the same. In his 1996 book, Carruthers listed them side by side: both women and men suffered mentally from fatigue, depression, irritability and reduced libido, and, on the physical side, from what he described as aging, aches and pains, sweating and flushing, and decreased sexual enjoyment (Carruthers 1996: 64–5). Andropause and menopause were similar but different, and clinicians wrestled with this paradox. On the one hand, they wanted to acknowledge the symptoms, because without symptoms there was no syndrome to diagnose or treat. On the other hand, men's fragile masculinity was still threatened by the diagnosis of a women's disease. What had to happen was that the subjective symptoms of andropause had to be clearly tied to an objective measurement of androgen levels, so that eventually the condition could be identified primarily by this quantitative assessment.

Controversy surrounded the measurement of testosterone levels in the blood and the meanings of those measurements. It was not until the 1960s that methods were developed to measure testosterone in human blood plasma; prior to this time, hormonal by-products and related gonadotropins excreted in the urine had to stand in as estimates. In the 1970s, radioimmunoassay techniques were employed in more sensitive tests of plasma hormone levels. The assays were complicated by the fact that testosterone circulated in the blood in several forms: free, bound to a protein called albumin, and bound to a different protein called sex-hormone-binding globulin. Free and albumin-bound testosterone made up the bioavailable testosterone; all three types taken together were considered total testosterone. Because androgen secretion was subject to circadian rhythms, the time of day when the blood was drawn also made a difference in the outcome of the test.

Clinicians varied in their opinions of the level at which testosterone (either total or bioavailable) ought to be considered sub-normal. Should the testosterone levels of middle-aged men be compared to those of men of comparable age or to the peak levels of men in their 20s? A group of urologists who chose the latter justified their decision as follows: 'Because there is no generally accepted threshold value of plasma testosterone for defining androgen deficiency, and in the absence of convincing evidence for an altered androgen requirement in older men, the normal range of testosterone levels in young males is suggested to be valid for older men as well' (Wald *et al.* 2006: 126). ISSAM recommended that 'abnormal' be defined as a testosterone level two standard deviations below the normal range of values for young men (Morales and Lunenfeld 2002: 76). As Steven Katz and Barbara Marshall have pointed out, the clinical concern was less about normality and more about functionality (Katz and Marshall 2004). Asymptomatic men might have very low testosterone levels that did not affect their sexual, physical or psychological functioning, but those men who complained of functional symptoms had their ailments validated by a low testosterone reading.

If low testosterone caused the symptoms of andropause, then replacing that testosterone should alleviate the symptoms. This simple equation was the basis of the 'therapeutic' test used in the 1940s: a patient was given testosterone injections for a period of several weeks, followed by placebo injections for several more weeks. If the patient experienced relief from his symptoms while on testosterone, but relapsed on the placebo, then his condition could be diagnosed as endocrine in origin (Watkins 2007b). By the end of the twentieth century, the more sensitive laboratory assays could directly measure the levels of testosterone in the blood and the results of the replacement therapy; the blood test provided an objective corroboration of the patient's subjective reporting of symptom relief.

Technology and testosterone: the gel

In 2000, another new delivery system for testosterone became available, accompanied by an aggressive marketing campaign that targeted both doctors and patients to raise awareness of low testosterone among aging men. Unimed Pharmaceuticals, a wholly-owned subsidiary of Solvay, won FDA approval for AndroGel, a clear colourless gel to be spread once a day on the upper arms, shoulders or abdomen. The approved labelling for AndroGel in 2000 listed the exact same indications as those for Androderm and Testoderm: primary or hypogonadotrophic hypogonadism due to either congenital or acquired causes. No mention was made of aging. The only difference between the patch and the gel was how the testosterone was applied to the skin. Building on the experience of TestoGel, a product available in France since the mid-1990s, Unimed hoped that the ease of the gel application, plus the lack of skin irritation caused by the patch, would convert current users of the patch and attract new users to its product (FDA 2000).[3]

Unimed bet right. AndroGel quickly garnered a large share of the American testosterone market. In 2002, almost one million prescriptions were dispensed, accounting for 54 percent of all the testosterone sold through retail pharmacies (Mehta 2009). That same year, AndroGel got a new competitor: Testim, produced by Auxilium Pharmaceuticals (FDA 2002). Although Testim, too, was approved only for the treatment of hypogonadism, Auxilium made explicit its intentions to go after the potentially enormous (and profitable) market of aging men.

Testim was Auxilium's first and only product for several years; in 2004, the company employed more than 100 salespeople to promote this product. In its annual report, the company told stockholders, 'Hypogonadism is a disorder that affects approximately 20% of the U.S. male population over age 50. We estimate there is a similar percentage of affected men in Europe' (Auxilium Pharmaceuticals 2004: 3). Two years later, it revised this estimate: '39% of men over 45 years of age have low testosterone (total testosterone levels below 300 ng/dL). According to the U.S. Census Bureau, there were 43.6 million men aged 45 to 84 in 2000, and these figures are expected to increase to 54.6 million by 2010. As a result, we expect to see an increase in the number of potential patients over the coming years' (Auxilium Pharmaceuticals 2006: 4).

In order to reach this largely untapped market, both clinicians and potential patients had to be educated about the significance of low testosterone. This education involved a rearticulation of the diagnosis of andropause. From the early 2000s, the defining marker would be a man's testosterone levels, as measured in nanograms per deciliter (ng/dL). Professional societies, such as ISSAM and the Endocrine Society, advised physicians to send their middle-aged and older male patients who exhibited any of the physical or psychological signs of andropause to the laboratory to have their blood hormone levels tested. A low number (generally, below 300 ng/dL) pointed to a diagnosis of late-onset hypogonadism (LOH), an endocrine deficiency that was the cause of the symptoms. This reduction of the clinical diagnosis to a quantitative measure accomplished two important objectives. First, the translation of andropause into late-onset hypogonadism, or low testosterone, reassured both (male) physicians and patients that men were not suffering from a woman's disease. Although changes in the conception and performance of masculinity had sanctioned men to look after their health, traditional values of manliness still differentiated between the two genders. Moreover, as Barbara Marshall has pointed out, a diagnosis of hypogonadism suggested 'a deficiency of androgens that result(ed) in demasculinization' with testosterone 'as the agent of re-masculinization' (Marshall 2009: 259). That is, these men could be seen as victims of a uniquely masculine disorder, not an age-related decline that could happen in members of either sex.

The second accomplishment of this transition from andropause to late-onset hypogonadism was that it allowed physicians to prescribe testosterone according to its labelled indications and, in so doing, to bill insurance companies for reimbursement for treatment of this genuine disorder.

Physicians had the right to prescribe any medication 'off-label'; however, if a physician could assign the diagnosis a valid code in the International Classification of Diseases (ICD) system, then a third-party payer might approve the prescription. The ICD-9 code 257.2 included the categories of hypogonadism for which Androderm, Testoderm, AndroGel and Testim were all indicated.

This strategy seemed to work: the number of testosterone prescriptions rose steadily through the 2000s. In 2008, almost three million prescriptions were filled in the United States, an increase of about 50 percent since 2003. AndroGel continued to dominate the market, with Testim a distant second (Mehta 2009). What is especially striking about this growth in testosterone replacement therapy is that it occurred *after* the largest-ever randomized controlled trial in women, the NIH-funded Women's Health Initiative (WHI), found that hormone replacement therapy in women was associated with increased risks of breast cancer, heart attacks, strokes and blood clots. As a result of this study, the prescription of oestrogen replacement declined rapidly (Watkins 2007a). While andropause advocates had used the alleged benefits of oestrogen in aging women in the 1990s to point to potentially similar health-promoting effects for testosterone in aging men, the corollary with regard to risks did not take hold among physicians or their patients, perhaps owing to the successful dissociation between andropause and menopause in the intervening years.

The Institute of Medicine report

Medical research funding agencies, however, did reconsider the issue of testosterone in light of the WHI. In November 2002, four months after the WHI results were released, the National Institute on Aging (NIA) and the National Cancer Institute (NCI) asked the Institute of Medicine (IOM) to evaluate the existing clinical research on testosterone therapy and aging and to recommend directions for future research in this arena. When the IOM released its report one year later, it based its recommendations on a few fundamental premises (Liverman and Blazer 2004). The committee agreed that testosterone should be used as a therapeutic intervention, not as a preventive measure, so that clinical studies should be conducted in subjects with obvious symptoms who had no other treatment options and might therefore benefit from treatment (as opposed to trials of testosterone in otherwise healthy men). Furthermore, the studies should be designed to evaluate testosterone's efficacy, that is, to establish whether or not replacement therapy had any clinically significant benefits, before going on to determine its long-term risks. These conditions were clearly a reaction to the WHI, which had enrolled only seemingly healthy participants in an effort to evaluate the long-term effects of HRT. With these stipulations in mind, the IOM committee recommended that clinical trials be conducted in men aged 65 and older with low testosterone levels (below the normal range of young adult males) and with at least one symptom in the following categories: weakness, frailty and disability; sexual dysfunction; cognitive dysfunction; impaired vitality, well-being and quality of life. The group recommended against a large-scale trial of the long-term risks and benefits of testosterone replacement therapy in aging men to match the Women's Health Initiative, at least until after the completion of initial short-term efficacy trials.

Medical journal articles once again emphasized the controversial aspects of testosterone therapy in the immediate wake of the IOM report, with titles such as 'Testosterone Treatment for the Aging Man: the Controversy', 'Andropause: Is Androgen Replacement Therapy Indicated for the Aging Male?,' and 'Testosterone in Older Men After the IOM Report: Where Do We Go from Here?' (Morales 2004; Hijazi and Cunningham 2005; Harman 2005). This literature lamented the IOM's recommendation against a large-scale trial. As S. M. Harman, of the Kronos Longevity Research Institute in Phoenix, put it:

> Despite nearly a half-century of research on aging and sex steroids in men, answers to key questions that would allow us to confidently assess risk:benefit ratios for androgen replacement in older men with partial androgen deficiency of aging men (PADAM) syndrome remains uncertain ... The US National Academies Institute of Medicine's recent report recommends that the National Institutes of Health support small efficacy trials aimed at treatment of androgen deficiency-related clinical conditions, but not a large, randomized trial to elucidate risk:benefit ratios. This recommendation, if adhered to, is likely to delay, rather than foster, progress in this important area.
>
> (Harman 2005: 124)

ISSAM, the International Society of Andrology, and the European Association of Urology revisited the recommendations they had made in 2002 about 'the investigation, treatment and monitoring of late-onset hypogonadism in males' and published the update simultaneously in four journals in 2005 (Nieschlag *et al.* 2005). By and large, the recommendations had not changed: in terms of diagnosis, men who presented with any of the acknowledged physical or psychological signs of possible hypogonadism should have a blood test to measure the level of testosterone. Those with the biochemical marker of low testosterone *and* the clinical marker of somatic or psychic symptoms earned the diagnosis of late-onset hypogonadism and could be treated with any of the available testosterone preparations on the market with the goal of attaining hormone levels in the normal range and relief from symptoms. In the absence of federally funded research on the risks of testosterone replacement therapy, clinicians would continue to prescribe it to their aging male patients who hoped to regain what were presented as lost aspects of their masculinity.

Conclusion

By 2008, there was general agreement in medicine that the measurement of blood testosterone levels could confirm the diagnosis of late-onset hypogonadism (LOH) in aging men. As Elianne Riska discusses elsewhere in this volume, LOH was cast as a health risk for aging men. Opinion was mixed on whether LOH was a treatable condition, but clinical advocates and pharmaceutical manufacturers of testosterone replacement therapy worked hard to promote it. Efforts to expand both the diagnosis of late-onset hypogonadism and the use of testosterone replacement therapy in aging men largely succeeded, as borne out by the steady increase in testosterone prescriptions over the past two decades.

Starting in the 1990s, the aging male appeared on the radar screen of physicians, thanks to a confluence of factors: concern than males of all ages were falling behind on a number of social axes, speculation about parallels between menopausal women and their male peers, and Viagra's erasure of taboos on talking about male sexual dysfunction. Acceptable performances of masculinity shifted and allowed more men to seek medical help to stave off the effects of aging. At the same time, traditional conceptions of manliness (i.e. not being a woman) were salvaged as doctors distanced andropause from menopause. They did so by converting it to a quantifiable entity. Following the trend toward greater reductionism in medicine – as, for example, in the measurement of blood pressure in diagnosing hypertension and cholesterol levels in prescribing statins – physicians transformed a previously qualitative syndrome into a quantitative diagnosis. In the twenty-first-century context of heightened awareness of men's health and proactive approaches to aging, this new spin on an old syndrome was just what the doctor ordered for the middle-aged man.

As historian of medicine Charles Rosenberg has observed, reductionism is tied to the concept of disease specificity, which 'in our culture ... is a fundamental aspect of the intellectual and moral legitimacy of disease' (Rosenberg 1989: 5). Male menopause regained medical legitimacy when it was reduced to late-onset hypogonadism in the medical literature; pharmaceutical manufacturers broadened its appeal for the general public by further simplifying it to Low T. This chapter has demonstrated that testosterone replacement therapy was a necessary, but not a sufficient, cause of increased medical attention to male aging in the late 1990s. Rather, medicalization, pharmaceuticalization and commercialization occurred within an assemblage of changing roles for men as health care consumers in American society, changing definitions and performances of masculinities, and changing expectations for medicine and pharmaceuticals in preventing diseases associated with growing old. The answer to the query posed in a 2002 article in *The New Yorker* magazine – is male menopause a question of medicine or marketing? – is not one or the other but both, at play within a fluid cultural matrix of assumptions about aging, masculinities and the biomedical enterprise.

Acknowledgements

I would like to thank Scott Podolsky and the editors of this volume for feedback on earlier drafts of this chapter. I am grateful to the National Endowment for the Humanities for a Fellowship in 2010–11 to support this project. Any views, findings, conclusions, or recommendations expressed in this publication do not necessarily reflect those of the National Endowment for the Humanities.

Notes

1 A search of PubMed, the international index of articles in biomedical journals, for the keywords male climacteric, male climacterium, male menopause, and andropause found just 10 articles in 1956–1969, 21 in the 1970s, 22 in the 1980s and 51 in the 1990s. For a closer look at the history of male menopause in the German context, see Hofer (2011, 2007). For a study of male menopause in Finland, see Vainionpaa and Topo 2005. For male menopause in Japan, see Sakai 2003.
2 My analysis is limited to mainstream medicine, but in the 1990s fringe practitioners of anti-aging medicine heavily promoted the use of testosterone and human growth hormone to prevent the effects of aging. For more on anti-aging medicine, see Weintraub 2010; Mykytyn 2010; Kampf and Botelho 2009.
3 The new testosterone gels were later found to cause virilization in women and children through secondary exposure; in 2009, the FDA required manufacturers to include a boxed warning on the prescribing information.

References

Alza Corporation (1996) *Annual Report*, filed 31 March 1997: www.secinfo.com (accessed Jan. 2011).
Auxilium Pharmaceuticals (2004) *Annual Report*, filed 15 April 2005: www.secinfo.com (accessed Feb. 2011).
Auxilium Pharmaceuticals (2006) *Annual Report*, filed 13 March 2007: www.secinfo.com (accessed Feb. 2011).
Carruthers, M. (1996) *Male Menopause: Restoring Vitality and Virility*, New York: HarperCollins.
Courtenay, W. H. (2000) 'Constructions of masculinity and their influence on men's well-being: A theory of gender and health', *Social Science and Medicine*, 50: 1385–1401.
FDA (1993) 'Testoderm NDA 19-762 approval package', Records of the Center for Drug Evaluation and Research, US Food and Drug Administration, Rockville, MD.
FDA (1995) 'Androderm NDA 20-489 approval package', Records of the Center for Drug Evaluation and Research, US Food and Drug Administration, Rockville, MD.
FDA (1997) 'Testoderm TTS NDA 20-791 approval package', Records of the Center for Drug Evaluation and Research, US Food and Drug Administration, Rockville, MD.
FDA (2000) 'Androgel NDA 21-015 approval package': http://www.accessdata.fda.gov/scripts/cder/drugsatfda/index.cfm (accessed Feb. 2011).

FDA (2002) 'Testim NDA 21-454 approval package': http://www.accessdata.fda.gov/scripts/cder/drugsatfda/index.cfm (accessed Feb. 2011).
Fishman, J. R. (2007) 'Making Viagra: From impotence to erectile dysfunction', in A. Tone and E. S. Watkins (eds), *Medicating Modern America: Prescription Drugs in History* (pp. 229–52), New York: New York University Press.
Gould, D. C., and Petty, R. (2000) 'The male menopause – does it exist?', *British Medical Journal*, 320: 858–60.
Gray, A., Berlin, J. A., McKinlay, J. B., and Longcope, C. (1991) 'An examination of research design effects on the association of testosterone and male aging: Results of a meta-analysis', *Journal of Clinical Epidemiology*, 44: 671–84.
Harman, S. M. (2005) 'Testosterone in older men after the IOM Report: Where do we go from here', *Climacteric*, 8: 124–35.
Hijazi, R. A., and Cunningham, G. R. (2005), 'Andropause: Is androgen replacement therapy indicated for the aging male?', *Annual Reviews in Medicine*, 56: 117–37.
Hofer, Hans Georg (2007), 'Medizin, Altern, Männlichkeit: Zur Kulturgeschichte des männlichen Klimakteriums', *Medizinhistorisches Journal*, 42: 210–45.
Hofer, Hans Georg (2011) 'Männer im kritischen Alter: Kurt Mendel und die Kontroverse über das männliche Klimakterium', *Der Urologe*, 50: 839–45.
ISSAM (1999) 'Mission statement', *The Aging Male*, 2: 6–7.
Kampf, A., and Botelho, L. A. (2009) 'Anti-aging and biomedicine: Critical studies on the pursuit of maintaining, revitalizing and enhancing aging bodies', *Medicine Studies*, 1: 187–95.
Katz, S., and Marshall, B. L. (2004) 'Is the functional "normal"? Aging, sexuality and the bio-marking of successful living', *History of the Human Sciences*, 17: 53–75.
Liverman, C., and Blazer, D. G. (eds) (2004) *Testosterone and Aging: Clinical Research Directions*, Washington, DC: National Academies Press.
Loe, M. (2004) *The Rise of Viagra: How the Little Blue Pill Changed Sex in America*, New York: New York University Press.
Lunenfeld, B. (1998) 'Aging male', *The Aging Male*, 1: 1–7.
Marshall, B. L. (2007) 'Climacteric redux? (Re)medicalizing the male menopause', *Men and Masculinities*, 9: 509–29.
Marshall, B. L. (2009) 'Rejuvenation's return: Anti-aging and re-masculinization in biomedical discourse on the "aging male"', *Medicine Studies*, 1: 249–65.
Matsumoto, A. M. (2002) 'Andropause: Clinical implications of the decline in serum testosterone levels with aging in men', *Journal of Gerontology: Medical Sciences*, 57A: M76–99.
Mehta, H. (2009) 'AndroGel (testosterone) BPCA drug use review': www.fda.gov/downloads/AdvisoryCommittees/CommitteesMeetingMaterials/PediatricAdvisoryCommittee/UCM166697.pdf (accessed Oct. 2010).
Morales, A. (2004) 'Testosterone treatment for the aging man: The controversy', *Current Urology Reports*, 5: 472–7.
Morales, A., and Lunenfeld, B. (2002) 'Investigation, treatment and monitoring of late-onset hypogonadism in males: Official recommendations of ISSAM', *The Aging Male*, 5: 74–86.
Mykytyn, C. E. (2010) 'A history of the future: The emergence of contemporary anti-ageing medicine', *Sociology of Health and Illness*, 32: 181–96.
Nieschlag, E., Swerdloff, R., Behre, H. M., Gooren, L. J., Kaufman, J. M., Legros, J. J., Lunenfeld, B., Morley, J. E., Schulman, C., Wang, C., Weidner, W., Wu, F. C.

(2005) 'Investigating, treatment and monitoring of late-onset hypogonadism in males', *The Aging Male*, 8: 56–8.
Orwoll, E. S. (2001) 'Equal time for the older male: Pathophysiology, evaluation, and management of male osteoporosis', *Annals of Long Term Care,* 9: 1–2.
Rosenberg, C. (1989) 'Disease in history: Frames and framers', *Milbank Quarterly,* 67 (suppl. 1): 1–15.
Sakai, Tomoko (2003), 'Narratives of *Dansei Konenki*: The indigenization of male menopause in contemporary Japan', *Undergraduate Research Journal for the Human Sciences*, 2: http://www.kon.org/urc/urc_research_journal2.html (accessed Oct. 2011).
Stengel, R. (1991) 'Bang the drum quietly', *Time* (8 July).
Tenover, J. L. (1998) 'Male hormone replacement therapy including "Andropause"', *Endocrinology and Metabolism Clinics*, 27: 969–87.
Vainionpaa, K. J., and Topo, P. (2005) 'The making of an ageing disease: The representation of the male menopause in Finnish medical literature', *Ageing and Society*, 25: 841–61.
Wald, M., Meacham, R. B., Ross, L. S., and Niederberger, C. S. (2006) 'Testosterone replacement therapy for older men', *Journal of Andrology*, 27: 126–32.
Watkins, E. S. (2007a) *The Estrogen Elixir: A History of Hormone Replacement Therapy in America*, Baltimore, MD: Johns Hopkins University Press.
Watkins, E. S. (2007b) 'The medicalisation of male menopause in America', *Social History of Medicine*, 20: 369–88.
Watkins, E. S. (2008) 'Medicine, masculinity, and the disappearance of male menopause in the 1950s', *Social History of Medicine*, 21: 329–44.
Weintraub, A. (2010) *Selling the Fountain of Youth: How the Anti-Aging Industry Made a Disease out of Getting Old – and Made Billions,* New York: Basic Books.
Weksler, M. E. (1995) 'Hormone replacement therapy for men: Has the time come?', *Geriatrics*, 50: 52–5.

3 'There is a person here'

Rethinking age(ing), gender and prostate cancer

Antje Kampf

This chapter explores the construction of the person within the discourses of prostate cancer.[1]

Issues around aging men diagnosed with prostate cancer, including its impact on their physiology, sexuality and identity, have only recently received sustained interest in the social sciences.[2] From a historical perspective, prostate cancer has remained under-researched throughout the twentieth century, even though definitions of masculinity shifted significantly during this period.

Social science studies have rightly emphasized the importance of recognizing the aging body as socially and culturally constituted (Calasanti 2008). Yet there seems to be a tendency to avoid the 'materiality' of aging bodies for fear of reducing age to biological decline and hence disempowering aged people. A parallel might be noted here with the earlier reticence of feminists to essentialize biological features of women that might serve to legitimize certain functions or social roles (see e.g. Hubbard 1992; Fausto-Sterling 2000). The issues of impairment and aging, central aspects of the prostate cancer experience, have been largely avoided, as has the issue of how identity is tied to the body (see also Meijer and Prins 1998; Wendell 1996; Shakespeare 1999).

In this chapter, I draw on feminist debates about the materiality of bodies to put men's bodies at centre stage, treating aging men's bodies as trajectories for wider issues of social status and roles. To this end, I explore issues around aging, gender and prostate cancer via an understanding of corporeality as the material condition of embodiment (cf. Csordas 1999). As Drew Leder has insisted, the body is 'at once a biological organism, a ground of personal identity, and a social construct' (1990: 99). These themes will be exemplified through an examination of the production of discourse concerning prostate cancer. I draw on a review of historical and contemporary clinical literature – using mainly examples from Germany and the European context, as well as an analysis of internet threads and observations from open-access prostate cancer support blogs. In doing so, I am guided by the desire to understand how bodies are lived in and shaped, how they are technically mediated and how they are 'experienced' in prostate cancer discourses. Drawing inspiration from theorists such as Scheper-Hughes, Lock, Mol and Law

(Scheper-Hughes and Lock 1987; Mol and Law 2004) who discern different types of bodies constructed in discourse, I review the history and analysis of prostate cancer through the lenses of (1) the aging body, (2) the sexual body, (3) the statistical body and (4) the social body. The chapter will start this investigation by illuminating the apparently most obvious body in prostate cancer debates, the aging body.

The aging body

The incidence of prostate cancer rises with increasing age so that, by age 70, studies suggest that about 70 percent of men have at least microscopic evidence of prostate cancers (Hoffman 2011). Despite an increasing diagnosis of prostate cancer in comparatively younger men in recent years, it is still considered a disease of aging men. Thus, the category of age is central in considering men's experience of prostate cancer, and in analysing biomedical practices and academic research related to it. The importance accorded age in these discourses is variable and at times contradictory. It plays a vital role with regards to therapeutic decisions, which consider not only the stage of the tumour and the general health of the man, but also his age. The effects of age on the efficacy of therapeutic interventions have been widely debated, as has (more recently) the issue of age within prevention and risk-management discourses. Until quite recently, older men have experienced 'contemporary invisibility' and marginalization in health organizational structures (Thompson 1995; Fleming 1999: 3–8; Calasanti 2008: 52–7), and this trend has extended to prostate cancer debates.

The relatively late emergence of debates about the prevention of prostate cancer in the second half of the twentieth century can be directly linked to its relationship with old age. The first major medical German textbook on gender and disease (Bürger 1960) does not mention prostate cancer in its general discussion on cancer statistics. The classic if controversial study by Erwin Liek (1934) on cancer prevention sidelined prostate cancer, even though discussing at length the relationship between age and cancer. And while by the late twentieth century the German Ministry of Health announced cancer as one of the major health targets, it left the issue of prostate cancer unexamined. Of course, over the course of the twentieth century, the definition of what constitutes an aging body in biological terms and in social roles has varied (Marshall and Katz 2002; Marshall 2011; Watkins this volume). Prominent, however, was the image of old age as something deficient, a view that prevailed until the 1970s (Michel 2006). Until the 1970s, state-sponsored health promotion (which included disease prevention) specifically for old people was minimal, a trend noted by academics in both the UK (Powell 2001) and Germany (Garms-Homolova 1991). This did not meaningfully shift until the emergence of special-interest groups, which focused on social relations rather than bodily functions as vital for good health in old age.

Age, in the medical debates, was a variable state, and sexuality and aging were not necessarily incompatible (Bloch 1909: 499). However, the main emphasis was on the age-related decline of libido and sexual function, resulting in men's desexualization – something which was perceived to be a 'natural' process (Marcuse 1927). As Magnus Hirschfeld, Germany's pre-eminent sexologist at the time, emphasized, this decline was accompanied by an increase in feminine characteristics (Hirschfeld 1926: 515, 352). This was not, however, believed to affect the morale of older men. Some of the medical sources seemed to endorse this account, dissociating sexual issues and age on the assumption that older people would have no real interest in sexual activity (Schirren 1966: 2098). This led, in part, to a disregard for the psychological effects of hormonal castration in cases of prostate cancer because those affected were 'mainly old and decrepit carcinoma patients' (Wildbolz 1952: 466), or rejection of older prostate cancer patients' wish for penis reconstruction for 'age-related reasons' (Vohl 1979).

Age thus functions as a normative category, which does not leave much room for considering how different ages and life stages may be associated with very specific stresses and thus may affect the life quality of men with prostate cancer. Nor does it leave room for individual life choices or strategies for coping with disease. The emphasis in the medical and state campaigns on the treatment of prostate cancer and in related academic discussions of bodies and patient identities is often firmly fixed on the life of the 'old cancer patient', rather than the life of 'the person with cancer' (Klotz 1997: 142; Deutsche Krebshilfe 2008: 56). This corresponds with what has been increasingly referred to as ageism in oncology, a set of cultural barriers and misconceptions which may result in differential access to services, therapy and clinical trials (see e.g. Yellen *et al.* 1994).

Recent critical gerontology has drawn attention to changing cultural discourses of aging and health which have differentiated between a relatively healthy 'Third Age' and a 'Fourth Age' of infirmity and decline (see also Higgs and McGowan in this volume; Gilleard and Higgs 2011; Baltes and Smith 2003). The influence of this distinction is evident, for example, in the growing debates about the use of Gynodian Depot (DHEA) and Hormone replacement therapies (HRT) for men diagnosed with prostate cancer that have been at the centre of anti-aging advocates' concerns to strengthen the vitality of the Third Age (for a critical discussion, see e.g. Kampf and Botelho 2009). Developments in screening, resulting in preclinical diagnosis and therapy, have increased the number of men living in a chronic disease state (Aronowitz 2009) and cancer survivorship (Bell and Kazanjian 2011). Noteworthy here is that the current trends shift the focus to younger men (above age 40 and below the threshold of 60 years of age) – those who are easier to target for lifestyle changes – despite a type of cancer that is usually very slow growing and infrequently the primary cause of death among older men. With the focus increasingly placed on younger men, aged men become marginalized within prostate cancer discourses.

The sexual body

I have suggested that the aged body has been (re)marginalized within prostate cancer discourses, a process which has had a direct bearing on the way in which attention has been given to the issue of sexuality. Given that the prostate is a gland that produces nourishing and protecting sperm fluid, it has a profound impact on male virility and sexuality – both of which are considered to be dominant markers of masculine identity. Yet the prostate's anatomical position and its concomitant relation with old age have meant that it has escaped notice in debates on male sexuality until recently. In the past decade, the impact of prostate cancer and prostate cancer therapy on idealized masculinity has attracted the interest of a number of researchers exploring its social (Oliffe 2005; Wassersug 2010; Asencio et al. 2009; Maliski et al. 2008) and historical dimensions (Kampf, 2009). This interest echoes the broader trend in aging studies and masculinity studies in exploring intersections of medical and cultural discourses on sexuality, masculinity and aging, culminating in recent work on Viagra and the treatment of impotence (see e.g. Marshall 2011).

A focus on the sexual body as central to masculine bodily norms has been cast as a recent phenomenon in prostate cancer history. However, it played its part in the early nosology and diagnosis of the disease. From the late nineteenth century onwards, the penis's use and abuse, and function and dysfunction, became a focus of attention in medical circles. Concerns were expressed about masturbation, sexual criminals, the prevalence of venereal disease infection and the perceived threats of homosexuals, all of which were believed to have implications for prostate health. Warnings were offered about the danger of an excess of sexual activity and the abuse of the prostate gland and/or the penis (including coitus interruptus) possibly leading to cancer in later life (Marcuse 1927: 256). These issues were tied up with the larger history of social hygiene, sexologists' growing interest in hermaphroditism and rejuvenation research.[3] Concern about the bodily norms of masculinity finally erupted within larger discussions about homophobia and concomitant fears about an 'emasculation' of politics and 'feminizing' of the state and 'unmanly men' in the decades before the First World War (zur Nieden 2005: 24).

All of this stood in stark contrast to the early twentieth-century 'German ideal of modern masculinity' which positioned the heterosexual, married 'sexually healthy functional" man as the norm, a figure who had well-balanced bodily structures, virility and sexual capability (Bloch 1909: 555). Male potency was constructed as central to a man's identity, his energy, courage and his will to work and live. As one writer of the time expressed it, 'In many cases, it is better to be dead than impotent' (Von Gyurkovechky 1897: 3).

The gendered dimensions of early diagnostics and therapy were not lost on at least some of these early physicians. For example, there are suggestions that it was undoubtedly embarrassment that held men back visiting physicians, particularly as the examination practice for prostate cancer's early detection involved bending down for a rectal examination (Haak 2002: 22). Some noted that prostatectomy would result in post-surgical stress or what one urologist termed a 'real mental disturbance' (Cholzhoff 1910: 652). In the main, however, the altered state of the body (and its normalized functionality) led to a disappearance of sexual meanings when the majority of doctors did not, however, unlike their male patients, connect men's identity with their sexual organs and corporeal features. Prostate cancer afflicts mainly elderly men, i.e. those who it was customarily believed no longer held sexuality as central to their bodies and male identity. A number of patients came to the clinics already at an advanced stage in the progress of the disease; they were in severe pain and had a typically short life expectancy after initial diagnosis (Blum and Rubritius 1928: 686). Often operations were performed less for curative than for palliative reasons, in order to slow down the growing destruction. While physiology was not expected to play any sexual role anymore, the 'man in the body' remained present in some of the case histories, where his socio-cultural role was acknowledged by listing his occupation and family status including the status of fatherhood.

With the more widely introduced use of prostatectomy in clinical practices after the 1940s, sources indicate that many men rejected any treatment for prostate cancer that entailed the possibility of impotency and a reduction of what they considered to be their quality of life (Klosterhalfen 1958: 680). Urologists have tended to downplay the number of patients with post-surgical erectile dysfunction and impotency, in order to persuade men to go ahead with the operation (Kubitschek 1994), indicating the importance of saving lives. The assumption of 'desexualisation' as a 'natural process' (Marshall 2006) has changed since the introduction of a (re)newed interest in the functional body (including functional sexuality). The onset of new biomedical and pharmacological technologies in the later part of the twentieth century to counteract age-related sexual decline (such as intra-cavernous injections, oral pharmacological medications, vacuum-pump devices, penis prosthesis, new nerve-sparing surgical techniques utilized clinically for localized prostate cancer) were meeting a rising demand created by the concomitant increase in self-help literature, internet networking and the use of other self-help forums.[4] Through these networks, aging men have demanded greater access to information on the relation between sexual function and the therapeutic options available to them. Doctors have catered to these needs by declaring the dys-appearance of sexuality a treatable disease, now termed 'erectile dysfunction' (see e.g. Watkins; Riska in this volume; Marshall and Katz 2002). At the same time, new diagnostic technologies since the 1990s have increased the trend of applying proactive therapy (such as oestrogen therapy) early in the course of the disease, producing the unwanted, but often unavoidable effect of emasculation.

Sexuality and the capacity for sexual practices and desires remain part of the embodied self, a situation that does not change for many men irrespective of age or health status, exemplified in various German online forum and network threads (Forum Prostatakrebs-bps 2008; Lifeline Forum Prostatakrebs 2006; NetDoktor Forum Prostata 2006). Sociological research here has documented men left facing a crisis of masculinity, yet at the same time stressing the opportunities of modifying normative ideals of male identity by opening up different notions of what sexuality entails (Kelly 2009; Oliffe 2005; Asencio et al. 2009).[5] Men's perspectives on sexuality and aging and living with prostate cancer is still, despite recent initiated quality-of-life-research (HAROW 2008), unexplored territory, at least in the German context. This difference between an apparent objective and subjective sexual body appears to collapse with the introduction of biomedical diagnostic technologies that identify bodies 'at risk' of cancer.

The statistical body (the body at risk)

Quantification of the human body and early detection testing technologies in medicine and cancer research have both become commonplace within biomedicine as a means of knowing bodies objectively (e.g. Pickstone 2011). This is also the case with prostate cancer. Questions typically arise about what exactly is prostate cancer and when it first appears, leading to predictions about its outcome, about when it stays benign or when it progresses to invasive cancer. Both aging and maleness itself have been thought to offer an inherent risk of acquiring prostate cancer (Kampf 2010). The diagnostic possibilities that have been introduced as part of a modern risk society (Beck 1992) play a decisive (albeit controversial) role in defining degrees and forms of risk and uncertainty and concurrent results on aging men which are embedded within and generated by the screening processes themselves (Howson 2001). A parallel can be found with breast cancer screening (Löwy 2007).

The tactile *feel* of the cancer marked the earliest ways of detecting it. Now, this low-tech rectal examination procedure, disliked by patients as well as physicians, has been extended by a dazzling array of early diagnostic tests and technologies (PSA, PSA kinectis, DNA biocytometry, biopsy, microarrays), out of which the PSA test – which measures the level of prostate-specific antigen in the blood – is perhaps still the most widely used. The PSA test has certainly become a function of 'instrumental rationality' (Kelleher 1994: 114) by facilitating a movement from uncertainties to relative certainties. However, the test masks a number of complex and unresolved issues within epidemiological debates. The test does not simply generate a biological marker that quantifies the presence of certain proteins within the male body, but is something that requires the expertise of an experienced 'reader' who can 'identify' the numbers and translate them into possible risk markers. As such, the test basically functions as a front-line detector only, making further diagnostic tests necessary. Refined diagnostic tests such as the newly introduced PSA kinetics produce equally ambivalent results, with multiple test systems in place and a built-in ambiguity about which classification system to use (Loeb 2009).

Despite the shortcomings, both in terms of diagnostic and early detection technology and of grade classification and prognosis, PSA testing has been adapted to include the concepts of active watching and watchful waiting: the idea is not simply to get a diagnostic result, but also to gain the basic values for the concurrent active monitoring of the statistical curve of the PSA and Gleason score values.[6] By so doing, the patient hopes he will reduce the risk of over-therapy and is granted the chance to decide when to start treatment (see also Deutsche Gesellschaft für Urologie e.V. 2009). The test, together with other forms of medical and self-scrutiny, may become an integral part of male aging.

Within medical circles, the PSA test is controversial,[7] leaving doctors and patients equally insecure (e.g. Caroll 2005). Men in a number of cases (at least on the internet forums) have asked their urologists whether the security they feel after testing negative should be instead be a worry (e.g. 'Klahei' 2005; 'Didi' 2005). However, the test remains a central tool in cancer progression diagnosis and, more importantly, men continue to use PSA results to manage insecurity (cf. Bell and Kazanjian 2011; Kampf 2010). Home-test kits, mathematical tables in health pamphlets and prostate-cancer risk calculators taken from the internet have all enabled men to correlate their own biometrical data and so make a 'certain' decision on how to proceed, and with which kind of therapy. With so many men having done the (PSA) tests secretly, there are controversies over studies, which are marred by opportunistic screenings (i.e. lacking men in control groups who have not yet done the test: cf. Wirth and Fröhner 2012). Mirroring Nikolas Rose's notion of the 'responsibility for the self to manage its present' (Rose 2007:134), the PSA test has gained new meaning in the trajectory on the graphs that men draw as they compile statistics in online support groups. Following the curving ups and downs of their blood and cell tests – not only do they follow the state of their bodily health on paper, but they also gain a prospective view into their future bodily integrity, making them anxiously await knowledge about their futures (e.g. 'HansiB' 2007; 'Hans76' 2007; 'Reinardo' 2007; 'Paul-Peter' 2007). An informal interview with a urologist at a university clinic in December 2008 confirms that a majority of patients who repeatedly visit the clinic rooms attend with self-drawn PSA charts for follow-up. The processes of the statistical bodies of men with prostate cancer reveal a paradox. On the one hand, the machinery of these tests transforms the stable body into an unpredictable pathological entity and volatile body. On the other hand, they serve as means to make their body predictable through these objective 'scores'. In addition, the quantified and objective nature of such data permits men to create distance: the cancer and its current presence in the body is not *felt* subjectively but detected objectively from the results of the PSA and Gleason scores. As one cancer veteran writes: 'it looks like I have the same cancer as six years ago' ('Reinardo' 2007). Objectifying the cancer may be an important coping strategy, and this is a question for future research. So too is the related question of social roles and social environments of men suffering from prostate cancer – the 'social body' to which I will turn now.

The social body

Illuminating the social bodies of men with prostate cancer requires that we probe men's structural and social ways of making sense of their disease, as these locate them in communities and social structures. While some studies have focused on the impact of stereotypical notions of male behaviour of not seeking help (Hale *et al.* 2007), a small number of studies (Broom 2005; Oliffe 2009) have begun to investigate how men with prostate cancer have organized themselves into 'communities *for* which they speak' (Rose 2007: 144–5), namely, cancer support groups and online social networks.[8] Compared to the politically proactive HIV/AIDS and breast cancer self-help groups, prostate cancer self-support groups have been less publicly visible and they have not engaged in any contested manner. Their increasing formation as part of a European online movement (Ligensa 2009) and at numerous local groups has been rather quiet.[9] Yet men have been engaging within the networks of the self-help groups and also in online knowledge networks and forums for emotional support living with the uncertainties of their prostate cancer diagnosis.[10]

While recent sociological literature has discussed whether cancer patients using the internet have been empowered to question medical decision-making processes (see e.g. Broom 2005; Ziebland *et al.* 2004), I focus here on the question of what kind of understanding is communicated. Men in the online networks go beyond the simple accumulation of information in a number of ways. They produce first-hand data collection on the course of their own disease and therapy history. They also practise knowledge as a 'human action' (Shapin and Schaffer 1985: 344) by pushing doctors into using specific medications discussed beforehand on the website threads. Men use the internet as an intermediary between the inconsistencies and uncertainty of medical disciplines and therapies that bridge radiologists, oncologists and urologists; they exchange their bodily profiles by leaving their biodata on the forum sites for others to see, compare or comment upon. They translate the biotechnology of diagnostic testing to create new networks and 'social worlds' whilst bloggers in the forum start to meet specifically in order to share and discuss their diagrams and charts. Some even think aloud about expanding their work and so produce combined data sets to offer as a 'service' to other bloggers ('Paul-Peter' 2007; 'Dieter' 2007; 'Reinardo' 2006; 'Winfried W' 2007). Engaging with the biotechnology, men transform diagnostic tools into communication and community-building devices. In all of this, men do not appear to dispute biomedical science as such. For the most part, their practices of knowledge production adhere to medical practices as the only way to save or at least extend their lives. Yet the threads of these men on the websites indicate that they have a different understanding of what medicine should do in situations of insecurity and doubt. They demand a clinical flexibility that allows for the inclusion of experiential knowledge.

A still under-researched topic in the relationship between the materiality of prostate cancer and the embodied self is how men's ill bodies are intertwined with social relations of family and economy (but see Kelly 2009). The 'social body' goes well beyond the internal and intimate relationships between objects and subjects. For example, bloggers insist that there are 'sociological changes' within prostate cancer discourse which ultimately have a bearing on society's economy, such as the trend of receiving ever-increasing numbers of requests for support from men who are still of working age. This trend challenges the still-dominant view that most men in prostate cancer care are already retired. Multiple blogs by daughters and wives can be found in the forums (e.g. 'KarinaH' 2009; 'Kathi1888' 2009; 'Merci62' 2009), a development which has instigated a second strand of self-help groups catering specifically to women and wives (cf. Bottorff *et al.* 2007). We know little of the generational impact: while the forums reveal quite a number of daughters inquiring for the state of their fathers' health, testifying to the (stereotypical) common notion of an ethic of care as a distinctively feminine attitude (cf. Gilligan 1993), I have not found yet a single entry from a son inquiring. Whether this mirrors an equally stereotypical notion of a dissociation of care (and the body?) that is culturally linked to masculinities has yet to be investigated (cf. Davidson in this volume). The issue of older prostate cancer patients as *fathers* (not solely in their reproductive role but perhaps more importantly in their social roles) and men's bodies intertwined with family health and income still awaits much needed future research.

Conclusion

The foregoing reflections have illustrated how four distinct yet interrelated bodies have become central to current analyses of prostate cancer and aging men. The normative category of age has been closely connected with the invisibility of male bodies, the disease itself and its course within medical practices. Assumptions about the connections between age, masculinity and sexuality have contributed to the continuing invisibility of the 'person' in discourses about prostate cancer, and its reduction to one possible aspect of self. Through the expansion of diagnostic screening and the central role played by statistics in modern neoliberal health policies and preventative medicine, chronic disease states have increasingly entered prostate cancer discourses. Biomedical diagnostics have lowered the age threshold of practices dealing with prostate cancer patients and have thereby (inadvertently) sidelined the needs of older men. Finally, I have argued that the social body, related to the social roles of aging men, is still the least interrogated aspect of scholarship on prostate cancer discourses.

I have tried to show that the unbecoming of a man as a consequence of the cancer itself, and by medical intervention, affects him in an anatomical sense, but also redefines how he conceptualizes his masculinity. This is an issue that requires proper consideration above and beyond the conceptual model of the normative male body. We have witnessed, in the last decade or so, an increase in sociological research on age discourses and male sexualities (cf. Marshall 2011) which might be brought to bear on understanding the medical and psychological aspects of experiencing prostate cancer and age discourses. Some research suggests that men do not necessarily reduce their identity to a reflection of their sexuality, and that for some men notions of sexual potency are quite fluid, and shift in relation to other bodily matters like their own mortality. However, the emphasis of research on aging men's bodies remains dominated by sexuality even if focused on its absence. But impairment of the lived body comes in many shades and meanings (cf. Kelly and Field 1996: 248) for men diagnosed with prostate cancer. It may be produced by the disease itself, or as a consequence of treatment. By probing into prostate cancer discourses, this chapter emphasizes the fact that a broader notion of bodily integrity should play a central role in research (cf. Williams 2006: 22).

This chapter thus encourages research that goes beyond the obvious connection with the sexual aspects of prostate cancer and calls for future research including long-term empirical study on how men deal with uncertainty and diagnostic advances. It also hopes to encourage scholarship investigating the important but so far neglected issue of how the social roles of men intersect with prostate cancer discourses. It furthermore calls for the equally vital even if challenging research into those men who have not engaged in social networks (on which much current research is necessarily based), those who have been left speechless by their disease experience (cf. 'Nick02' 2009).

In all these cases, 'there is a person here' who comes with a (bodily) complexity which marks and defines what it is to be an aging man with prostate cancer.

Acknowledgements

Earlier versions of this chapter were presented at the International Conference of the Society for Medical Anthropology of the American Anthropological Association at Yale University, and at the Conférence scientifique du MÉOS (Médicament comme objet social) at the Université de Montréal both in 2009. I would like to thank participants for helpful comments. I am grateful to the DAAD for a grant to support this project.

Notes

1 The quotation in the title is taken from Breen et al. 2001.
2 Specifically social science studies have begun to critically follow up on modern biomedical diagnostic and therapeutic possibilities for fighting prostate cancer, exploring their impact on aging men's bodies, lives, their social place (e.g. Gray et al. 2002; Oliffe 2005; Broom 2004; Wall and Kristjanson 2005; Nicholas 2000; Faulkner 2008) and psychological effects (cf. Kelly 2009; Hale et al. 2007). This new focus corresponds with a similar recent trend to investigate the historical (Hofer 2007; Watkins 2008) and sociological biomedical conceptualization of aging male bodies (e.g. Rosenfeld and Faircloth 2006; Katz and Marshall 2004; Marshall 2011; Petersen 1998).
3 While the rejuvenating effect of castration in cases of prostate hyperthrophy and its ameliorative effect on overall health was noted, it was not connected to issues of sexual performance.
4 Most technology studies suggest that it is never a one-way process of meeting pre-existing needs, but those needs and desires are often at least partially created by availability of technologies. However, in this instance, physicians' first priority was to get rid of the tumour, nerve sparing technology.
5 This vital research is, however, still based on small empirical base.
6 'Watchful waiting' (WW) has been introduced for older patients (above 65 years of age) and 'active surveillance' (AS) entailing curative therapy specifically for younger patients. The concept does not come without debate, given that in the USA few health care professionals recommend WW or AS as viable options; however, this strategy has been endorsed in other localities by the local urology association (e.g. Germany).
7 In 2011, an American expert panel advised against screening healthy men; in Germany and in Scandinavia, the test while still controversial has still been more favourably received (cf. Wirth and Fröhner 2012).
8 The introduction and structure of self-help organization and movement is not part of this paper but is increasingly gaining attention stemming predominantly from social science studies perspectives (e.g. Rabeharisoa and Callon 2008).
9 By comparison to the publicly more outspoken American-based 'UsTOO' online support network for prostate cancer. A discussion on these socio-cultural differences – while interesting – is beyond the scope of this paper.
10 While not constituting the majority of internet users, German studies have confirmed American trends suggesting that men from older age groups (i.e. those over 50 years old) are increasingly using the web – with men aged 60 and older more likely to do so than women in the same age group ((N)onliner Atlas 2011: 44).

References

Aronowitz, R. A. (2009) 'The converged experience of risk and disease', *Milbank Quarterly*, 87: 417–42.

Asencio, M., Blank, T., Descartes, L., and Crawford, A. (2009) 'The prospect of prostate cancer: A challenge for gay men's sexualities as they age', *Sexuality Research and Social Policy*, 6: 38–51.

Baltes, P. B., and Smith, J. (2003) 'New frontiers in the future of aging: From successful aging of the young old to the dilemmas of the fourth age', *Gerontology*, 49: 123–35.

Beck, U. (1992) *Risk Society: Towards a New Modernity*, New Delhi: Sage.

Bell, K., and Kazanjian, A. (2011) 'PSA testing: Molecular technologies and men's experience of prostate cancer survivorship', *Health, Risk and Society*, 13: 183–96.
Bloch, I. (1909) *Das Sexualleben unserer Zeit*, Berlin: Louis Marcus.
Blum, V., and Rubritius, H. (1928) 'Die Erkrankungen der Prostata', in A. Lichtenberg, F. Völcker and H. Wildbolz (eds), *Spezielle Urologie, Dritter Teil: Erkrankungen der Harnleiter, der Blase, Harnröhre, Samenblase, Prostata, des Hodens und Samenstranges und der Scheidenhäute, Scrotum; Gynäkologische Urologie* (pp. 634–688), Berlin: Springer.
Bottorf, J., Oliffe, J. L., Halpin, M., Phillips, M., McLean, G., and Mroz, L. (2007) 'Women and prostate cancer support groups', *Social Science and Medicine*, 66: 1217–27.
Breen, M. S., Blumenfeld, W. J., Baer, S., Brookey, R. L., Hall, L, Kirby, V., Miller, D. H., Shail, R., and Wilson, N. (2001) 'Introduction to "There is a Person Here": An interview with Judith Butler', *International Journal of Sexuality and Gender Studies*, 6: 7–20.
Broom, A. (2004) 'Prostate cancer and masculinity in Australian society: A case of stolen identity?', *International Journal of Men's Health*, 3: 73–91.
Broom, A. (2005) 'Virtually he@lthy: The impact of internet use on disease experience and the doctor–patient relationship', *Qualitative Health Research*, 15: 325–45.
Bürger, M. (1960) *Altern und Krankheit als Problem der Biomorphose*, Leipzig: Thieme.
Calasanti, T. (2008) 'A feminist confronts ageism', *Journal of Aging Studies*, 22: 52–7.
Carroll, P. R. (2005) 'Early stage prostate cancer – do we have a problem with over-detection, overtreatment or both?', *Journal of Urology*, 173: 1061–2.
Cholzhoff, B. N. (1910) 'Über Operationen beim Diffusen Krebs des Männlichen Gliedes', *Zeitschrift für Urologie*, 4: 649–59.
Csordas, T. (1999) 'Embodiment and cultural phenomenology', in G. Weiss and H. F. Haber (eds), *Perspectives on Embodiment: The Intersections of Nature and Culture* (pp. 143–162), London: Routledge.
Deutsche Gesellschaft für Urologie e.V. (2009) 'Europäische Studie: 20 Prozent weniger Prostatakrebstote dank PSA-Screening': http://www.urologenportal.de/944.html (accessed April 2009).
Deutsche Krebshilfe (2008) *Blaue Broschüre: Prostatakrebs*, Bonn: Deutsche Krebshilfe.
'Didi' (2005) 'Chat protocol "Hauptsache Gesund: Prostata", on air March 3, 2005': http://chat.mdr.de (accessed March 2008: the specific link for this protocol has since been deleted; the author has a copy of the protocol).
'Dieter' (2007) 'Feinnadel-Aspirationsbiopsie (3)': http://forum.prostatakrebs-bps.de/showthread.php?t=1874 (accessed April 2009).
Faulkner, A. (2008) *Medical Technology into Healthcare and Society: A Sociology of Devices, Innovation and Governance*, Basingstoke: Palgrave Macmillan.
Fausto-Sterling, A. (2000) *Sexing the Body: Gender Politics and the Construction of Sexuality*, New York: Basic Books.
Fleming, A. A. (1999) 'Older men in contemporary discourses on ageing: Absent bodies and invisible lives', *Nursing Inquiry*, 6: 3–8.
Forum Prostatakrebs-bps (2008) 'Prostatakrebs-Diskussionsforum': http://forum.prostatakrebs-bps.de (accessed March 2008).
Garms-Homolova, V. (1991) 'Prävention und Prophylaxe bei alten Menschen in der Bundesrepublik', in T. Elkeles, T. Niehoff, R. Rosenbrock and F. Schneider

(eds), *Prävention und Prophylaxe: Theorie und Praxis eines gesundheitspolitischen Grundmotivs in zwei deutschen Staaten 1949–1990* (pp. 319–37), Berlin: Edition Sigma.

Gilleard, C., and Higgs, P. F. (2011) 'Ageing abjection and embodiment in the Fourth Age', *Journal of Ageing Studies*, 25: 135–42.

Gilligan, C. (1993) *An Ethic of Care. Feminist and Interdisciplinary Perspectives*, New York and London: Routledge.

Gray, R., Fitch, M., Fergus, K., Mykhalovskiy, E., and Church, K. (2002) 'Hegemonic masculinity and the experience of prostate cancer: A narrative approach', *Journal of Aging and Identity*, 7: 43–62.

Haak, J. (2002) 'Der unbehandelte Mann', *Berliner Zeitung* (2 Oct.), 22.

Hale, S., Grogan, S., and Willott, S. (2007) 'Patterns of self-referral in men with symptoms of prostate disease', *British Journal of Health Psychology*, 12: 403–19.

'Hans76' (2007) 'Feinnadel-Aspirationsbiopsie (3)': http://forum.prostatakrebs-bps.de/showthread.php?t=1874 (accessed April 2009).

'HansiB' (2007) 'Feinnadel-Aspirationsbiopsie (3)': http://forum.prostatakrebs-bps.de/showthread.php?t=1874 (accessed April 2009).

HAROW (2008) 'Info 01/08': http://www.harow.de/html/img/pool/newsletter01.pdf (accessed April 2009).

Hirschfeld, M. (1926) *Geschlechtskunde*, vol. 1, *Die Körperseelischen Grundlagen*, Stuttgart: Julius Püttmann.

Hofer, H. G. (2007) 'Medizin, Altern, Männlichkeit: Zur Kulturgeschichte des Männlichen Klimakteriums', *Medizinhistorisches Journal*, 42: 210–245.

Hoffman, R. (2011) 'Screening for prostate cancer', *New England Journal of Medicine*, 365: 2013–19.

Howson, A. (2001) 'Locating uncertainties in cervical screening', *Health, Risk and Society*, 3: 167–79.

Hubbard, R (1992) *The Politics of Women's Biology*, 2nd edn, New Brunswick, NJ: Rutgers University Press.

Kampf, A. (2009) 'The absence of Adam: Prostate cancer and male identity', in J. Powell and T. Gilbert (eds), *Aging and Identity: A Postmodern Dialogue* (pp. 29–43), New York: Nova Science Publishers.

Kampf, A. (2010) '"The risk of age"? Early detection test, prostate cancer and technologies of self', *Journal of Aging Studies*, 24: 325–34.

Kampf, A., and Botelho, L. (2009) 'Anti-Aging and biomedicine: Bodies, gender, and the pursuit of longevity', *Medicine Studies: An International Journal for History, Philosophy, and Ethics of Medicine and Allied Sciences*, 1: 187–95.

'KarinaH' (2009) 'Sind Metastasen behandelbar?': http://forum.prostatakrebs-bps.de/showthread.php?t=4992 (accessed April 2009).

'Kathi1888' (2009) 'Zometa Nebenwirkungen': http://forum.prostatakrebs-bps.de/showthread.php?t=4725&page=2 (accessed April 2009).

Katz, S., and Marshall, B. (2004) 'Is the functional "normal"? Aging, sexuality and the bio-marking of successful living', *History of the Human Sciences*, 17: 53–75.

Kelleher, D. (1994) 'Self-help groups and medicine', in J. Gabe, D. Kelleher and G. Williams (eds), *Challenging Medicine* (pp. 104–17), London: Routledge.

Kelly, D. (2009) 'Changed men: The embodied impact of prostate cancer', *Qualitative Health Research*, 19: 151–63.

Kelly, M., and Field, D. (1996) 'Medical sociology, chronic illness and the body', *Sociology of Health and Illness*, 18: 241–57.

'Klahei' (2005) 'Chat protocol "Hauptsache Gesund: Prostata", on air March 3, 2005': http://chat.mdr.de (accessed March 2008: the specific link for this protocol has since been deleted; the author has a copy of the protocol).
Klosterhalfen, H. (1958) 'Betrachtungen zur Behandlung des Prostatakarzinoms', *Zeitschrift für Urologie*, 11: 680–9.
Klotz, T. (1997) 'Prävention von Krebskrankheiten', in K. Hurrelmann, T. Klotz, and J. Haisch (eds), *Lehrbuch Prävention und Gesundheitsförderung: Lehrbuch Gesundheitswissenschaften* (pp. 141–54), Berne: Hans Huber.
Kubitschek, J. (1994) 'Streit um die Prostata', *Focus*, 19: 148–58.
Leder, D. (1990) *The Absent Body*, Chicago: Chicago University Press.
Liek, E. (1934) *Der Kampf gegen den Krebs*, Munich: J. F. Lehmanns Verlag.
Lifeline Forum Prostatakrebs (2006) 'Chat protocol Expertenrat Prostatakrebs': http://www.lifeline.de/cda/forum/actionViewBoard.html?page=1&board=82&sortT=1 (accessed March 2008).
Ligensa, C. (2007) 'Europa Uomo Patiententag', *BPS Magazin*, 3: 9–10.
Loeb, S. (2009) 'Prostate cancer: Is PSA velocity useful?', *Nature Reviews Urology*, 6: 305–6.
Löwy, I. (2007) 'Breast cancer and the "materiality of risk": The rise of morphological prediction', *Bulletin of the History of Medicine*, 81: 241–66.
Maliski, S. L., Rivera, S., Connor, S., Lopez, G., and Litwin, M. S. (2008) 'Renegotiating masculine identity after prostate cancer treatment', *Qualitative Health Research*, 18: 1609–20.
Marcuse, M. (ed.) (1927) *Die Ehe: Ihre Physiologie, Psychologie, Hygiene und Eugenik. Ein Biologisches Ehebuch*, Berlin: Marcus & Weber.
Marshall, B. (2006) 'The new virility: Viagra, male aging and sexual function', *Sexualities*, 9: 345–62.
Marshall, B. (2011) 'The graying of "sexual health": A critical research agenda', *Canadian Review of Sociology*, 48: 390–413.
Marshall, B., and Katz, S. (2002) 'Forever functional: Sexual fitness and the ageing male body', *Body and Society*, 8: 43–70.
Meijer, I. C., and Prins, B. (1998) 'How bodies come to matter: An interview with Judith Butler', *Signs*, 23: 275–86.
'Merci62' (2009) 'Probleme im fortgeschrittenen Stadium': http://forum.prostatakrebs-bps.de/showthread.php?t=4822 (accessed April 2009).
Michel, B. (2006) 'Health promotion and prevention in old age: A discourse analysis from the beginning of the 19th century up to present times', unpublished thesis, Universitätsmedizin Berlin.
Mol, A., and Law, L. (2004) 'Embodied action, enacted bodies: The example of hypoglycaemia', *Body and Society*, 10: 43–62.
NetDoktor Forum Prostata (2006) 'Chatprotocol "Impotenz nach Prostatakrebs"': http://www.netdoktor.de/search/results?query=Impotenz+nach+prostatakrebs (accessed March 2008).
Nicholas, D. (2000) 'Men, masculinity and cancer risk-factor behaviours: Early detection and psychosocial adaptation', *Journal of American College Health*, 49: 27–33.
'Nick02' (2009) 'Frage an Daniel Schmidt': http://forum.prostatakrebs-bps.de/showthread.php?t=5014 (accessed April 2009).
(N)onliner Atlas (2011) 'Internetnutzung von Frauen und Männern in Deutschland 2011': http://www.nonliner-atlas.de (accessed Feb. 2012).

Oliffe, J. L. (2005) 'Constructions of masculinity following prostatectomy-induced impotence', *Social Science and Medicine*, 60: 2249–59.
Oliffe, J. L. (2009) 'Health behaviors, prostate cancer and masculinities: A life course perspective', *Men and Masculinities*, 11: 346–66.
'Paul-Peter' (2007) 'Feinnadel-Aspirationsbiopsie (3)': http://forum.prostatakrebs-bps.de/showthread.php?t=1874 (accessed April 2009).
Petersen, A. (1998) *Unmasking the Masculine: 'Men' and 'Identity' in a Sceptical Age*, London: Sage.
Pickstone, J. V. (2011) 'A brief introduction to ways of knowing and ways of working', *History of Science*, 49: 235–45.
Powell, J. (2001) 'Theorizing gerontology: The case of old age, professional power, and social policy in the United Kingdom', *Journal of Aging and Identity*, 6: 117–35.
Rabeharisoa, A. V., and Callon, M. (2008) 'The growing engagement of emergent concerned groups in political and economic life: Lessons from the French Association of neuromuscular disease patients', *Science, Technology and Human Values*, 33: 230–61.
'Reinardo' (2006) 'Feinnadel-Aspirationsbiopsie (3)': http://forum.prostatakrebs-bps.de/showthread.php?t=1874 (accessed April 2009).
'Reinardo' (2007) 'Feinnadel-Aspirationsbiopsie (3)': http://forum.prostatakrebs-bps.de/showthread.php?t=1874 (accessed April 2009).
Rose, N. (2007) *The Politics of Life itself*, Princeton, NJ, and Oxford: Princeton University Press.
Rosenfeld, D., and Faircloth, C. (eds) (2006) *Medicalised Masculinities*, Philadelphia, PA: Temple University Press.
Scheper-Hughes, N., and Lock, M. (1987) 'The mindful body: A prolegomenon to future work in medical anthropology', *Medical Anthropology Quarterly*, 1: 6–41.
Schirren, C. (1966) 'Fragen aus der Praxis', *Deutsche Medizinische Wochenschrift*, 91: 46.
Shakespeare, T. (1999) 'The sexual politics of disabled masculinity', *Sexuality and Disability*, 17: 53–64.
Shapin, S., and Schaffner S. (1985) *Natural Philosophy in the Scientific Revolution, Leviathan and the Air Pump: Hobbes, Boyle, and the Experimental Life*, Princeton, NJ: Princeton University Press.
Thompson, E. (ed.) (1995) *Older Men's Lives*, Thousand Oaks, CA: Sage.
Vohl, M. (1979) 'Fortschritte im Erkennen und Behandeln von Impotenz', unpublished thesis, Universität Hannover.
Von Gyurkovechky, V. G. V. (1897) *Pathologie und Therapie der Männlichen Impotenz*, 2nd (expanded) edn, Vienna and Leipzig: Urban & Schwarzenberg.
Wall, D., and Kristjanson, L. (2005) 'Men, culture and hegemonic masculinity: Understanding the experience of prostate cancer', *Nursing Inquiry*, 12: 87–97.
Wassersug, R. J. (2010) 'The language of emasculation: Implications for cancer patients', *International Journal of Men's Health*, 9: 3–25.
Watkins, E. (2008) 'Medicine, masculinity, and the disappearance of the male menopause in the 1950s', *Social History of Medicine*, 2: 1–16.
Wendell, S. (1996) *The Rejected Body: Feminist Philosophical Reflections on Disability*, London: Routledge.
Wildbolz, E. (1952) *Lehrbuch der Urologie und der chirurgischen Krankheiten der männlichen Geschlechtsorgane*, Berlin: Springer.

Williams, S. (2006) 'Medical sociology and the biological body: Where are we now and where do we go from here?', *Health: An Interdisciplinary Journal for the Social Study of Health, Illness and Medicine*, 10: 5–30.

'Winfried W.' (2007) 'Feinnadel-Aspirationsbiopsie (3)': http://forum.prostatakrebs-bps.de/showthread.php?t=1874 (accessed April 2009).

Wirth, N., and Fröhner, M. (2012) 'Für und Wider des Prostatakarzinomscreenings', Ärztezeitung.de: http://www.aerztezeitung.de/medizin/krankheiten/krebs/prostata krebs/article/800632/prostatakrebs-jaehrlicher-psa-test-senkt-sterberate-nicht.html (accessed Jan. 2012).

Yellen, S. B, Cella, D., and Leslie, W. T. (1994) 'Age and clinical decision making in oncology patients', *Journal of the National Cancer Institute*, 86: 1766–70.

Ziebland, S., Chapple, A., Dumelow, C., Evans, J., Prinjha, S., and Rozmovits, L. (2004) 'How the internet affects patient's experience of cancer: a qualitative study', *British Medical Journal*, 328: 564–70.

zur Nieden, S. (ed.) (2005) *Homosexualität und Staatsräson:* Männlichkeit, Homophobie und Politik in Deutschland, *1900–1945,* New York and Frankfurt: Campus.

Part II
Scientific and health discourses on aging men

4 Aging men

Resisting and endorsing medicalization

Elianne Riska

For almost forty years the concept of medicalization has been used to characterize the different agents influencing the definition of medical problems and the kind of bodies, behaviours and life events included in such definitions. Research on this topic has mainly looked at women's bodies and women's health; only recently has the analytical tool of medicalization been applied to men's bodies and men's health (Rosenfeld and Faircloth 2006). This chapter will look at the increasing tendency to medicalize men's health in general and the health of aging men in particular. The argument presented in this chapter is that men's health has been medicalized in a way different from the process of medicalization of women's health. One reason for this is that public discourse and public health discourse have conceptualized 'men's health' mainly in cultural terms and interpreted men's health behaviour as a cultural affirmation of the masculine script. The cultural approach is a remnant of the sex-role theory that in the 1950s and 1960s was a mainstream approach to explaining the acquisition of a female or male sex identity and sex role. Early feminist research and theorizing on 'women's health' as a specific field of research challenged the sex-role theory of health and health behaviour. In fact, the field of women's health and the women's health movement were central components in challenging not only the biological explanations of sex and gender but also mainstream sociological theories on the family and biomedical conceptions of women's body and health (Fee 1977). Such a critique has emerged much later concerning men's health and a number of important contributions have emerged during the past fifteen years (e.g. Sabo and Gordon 1995; Courtenay 2000; Broom and Tovey 2010; Oliffe 2006). Yet men's health as a specific field of study is still undertheorized, which has had implications for how aging men's health has been described and understood.

This chapter suggests that the current cultural approach makes aging men vulnerable to medicalization in two ways: to a medicalization of their cultural identity as men and to a naturalization or biologization of their health and bodies. This will be illuminated in three ways in this chapter. The first section presents the theories on medicalization, basic assumptions and arguments, and its use as a theoretical framework for understanding aging men's health. The theoretical perspectives on the medicalization argument will be exemplified in the second section. This section will look at two current scientific discourses on men's health that illustrate both men's resistance to and endorsement of a medicalization of aging. The first case concerns war veterans' views of the medical diagnosis of combat-related PTSD (post-traumatic stress disorder). The psychiatric label PTSD is a challenge to masculine values – self-reliance and remaining in control. As will be shown, war veterans' acceptance or rejection of the diagnosis as a shared disorder have been related to the context of the war. The second case deals with the tacit endorsement among aging men of the medicalization of androgen deficiency and the related testosterone-deficiency syndrome (TDS) and erectile dysfunction (ED).

The third section will compare how men have dealt with the labels of PTSD and TDS/ED. Both labels contain notions of a loss of the masculine self and the experience of an enfeebled masculinity. The physical symptoms of fatigue, low libido and impotence related to PTSD and TDS/ED encapsulate the demasculinizing effects of aging. The comparison will show that the psychiatric label of PTSD has resulted in more challenges and collective redefinitions by war veterans than has the endocrinologically constituted aging male body offered by the TDS/ED labels. The conclusion will point to the weaknesses of the theoretical perspectives – based on a cultural theory of masculinity – on aging men, and men's health studies in general.

Medicalization of men's health

The term *medicalization* was introduced into sociology in the early 1970s (Zola 1972). The term has been used to indicate the definitional process whereby a certain life condition, social behaviour or social status has been delegated to the medical profession for treatment and control.

Over the years the forces behind the 'medicalizing processes' have been given new interpretations. The first to give the term a special meaning were feminist scholars, who argued that women were the primary targets of the expanding jurisdiction of medicine (Riska 2003). The second influence on the debate came from critics in the 1980s who argued that among women there was resistance to medicalization (e.g. Riessman 1983). In the 1990s, the new field of sociology of the body pointed to the complex definitional process of the cultural and biological aspects of the body and illnesses in the process of medicalization (Lupton 1997). In the mid-2000s, Conrad (2005, 2007) conceptualized the different stages of the medicalization process with the phrase 'the shifting engines of medicalization'. He pointed to consumers and the pharmaceutical industry as the new agents in the process. The term *pharmaceuticalization* (Abraham 2010; Williams *et al.* 2011) has more recently been introduced to illustrate the global cultural and economic power of the international pharmaceutical companies in medicalizing symptoms and in creating a market for new drugs. Others (Fox and Ward 2008) have introduced the phrase 'pharmaceuticalization of daily life' to signal the link between the macro and micro levels in the drug industry's influence on the private sphere.

A recent proponent for a new interpretation is represented by Clarke and her research group (2003, 2010), who have argued that the term *biomedicalization* highlights a new, qualitative change in the medicalization process. Their focus is on knowledge-making practices, especially how the body is discursively constituted through biomedical knowledge and practices. Their central argument is that the new technoscience and biomedical corporate enterprise influence not only how medicine is practised but also how technoscientific discourses penetrate the public discourse. Clarke and her colleagues argue that biomedicalization has reconstructed the boundaries between the material body and social identity so that medical interventions in the form of 'technologies of the body' enable an enhancement of a certain type of revered notion of the self (e.g. a sexually potent person) and the creation of technoscientific identities (Clarke *et al.* 2003: 184).

The scholarly debate summarized above has ranged from a social interactionist, to a social constructionist, to a post-structural perspective. In this theorizing, men's health has often been forgotten. It has been tacitly assumed that issues examined by the sociological terms 'gender and health' and 'medicalization' concern mainly women. The next two sections will examine two areas of research that have explicitly looked at the medicalization of aging men's health, masculinity and the power of medicine: the mental health of war veterans and the sexual health of aging men.

Confronting medicalization: war, mental health and masculinity

Much of the traditional and feminist research on mental health deals mainly with women's health (Chesler 1989). The need to look at gender and mental health and the gendered construction of mental health has been pointed out in historical and contemporary studies (Chesler 1989; Lunbeck 1998; Busfield 1996; Kempner 2006). An area specifically concerned with men's mental health problems is related to the long-term effect of combat experience on men's mental health. Much of this literature has been gender-blind in the sense that it is taken for granted that it is about a health issue that affects men and that the term 'war veteran' signifies a man.

Men's collective reaction to the health impact of different types of war suggests that masculinity is made and remade at the intersection of war and culture. As several scholars have noted, war and masculinity have been mutually constitutive (Jeffords 1989, 1994; Karner 1995; Mosse 2000; Hutchings 2008; Kilshaw 2008a, 2008b). The ideals of masculinity are seen as essential and functional for men's participation in combat: aggression, physical strength, emotional toughness. These characteristics have also been defined as hegemonic masculinity, a concept that rests on a hierarchical distinction not only between masculinity and femininity but also between different types of masculinity (Connell and Messerschmidt 2005).

War trauma has emerged as a special diagnostic category and was given the diagnostic label post-traumatic stress disorder (PTSD) in the third *Diagnostic and Statistical Manual of Mental Disorders* (DSM-III) in 1980. It is included in the current fourth version (DSM-IV, published in 2000). The cultural and social embeddedness of this category has been pointed out by many researchers (Young 1995: 5; Bracken 2001: 741). Furthermore, scholars have pointed to the gender aspect of the diagnosis and noted that 'PTSD has not been investigated in terms of how men as men experience it' (Karner 2008: 85). In most psychiatric research PTSD has been presented as a gender-neutral concept. As the next section will show, its use as a way of processing war veterans' mental health complaints generally carries with it a notion of injured or threatened masculinity.

Two social structures – the military and the profession of psychiatry – serve as the counter parties with which war veterans have to negotiate their illness claims. Psychiatry as a profession and scientific paradigm is the formal agent in the process of acknowledgement of the medical legitimacy of the complaints. The military as an institution has in many wars, especially beginning with the Korean War, collaborated in preventive ways with the profession of psychiatry in order to maintain a functional military personnel. For veterans this collaboration has at times been controversial, because the military culture stands for values that define mental problems as a sign of weakness and embodied femininity (Mosse 2000; Hutchings 2008; Kilshaw 2008a). Hence, mental health problems have not only the stigma they have in the general society but war veterans become doubly stigmatized.

Mental health symptoms brought about by war experiences have been a topic of both resistance and contestation among the war veterans themselves. In this area the term *medicalization* can be used as an analytical tool for understanding how war veterans have defined long-lasting mental health problems related to their past involvement in combat.

The process of lay involvement in the medicalization of a symptom has been called the 'diagnosis negotiation' and 'politics of definitions' (Zavestoski *et al.* 2004: 162). The diagnosis negotiation is a central feature of those diseases that have contested symptoms. Brown and his colleagues (2000: 236) have defined 'contested illnesses' as diseases and conditions that involve major scientific disputes and public debates over the medical legitimacy of environmental causes. This dispute generally involves conflicting claims about whether a symptom has a 'real' organic cause within the framework of existing biomedicine or whether the symptoms have an individual and idiosyncratic causation.

Medicalization of war veterans' health symptoms: war and mental health

The research literature on war veterans' mental health profile includes the mental health impact of the following eight wars: World War I, World War II, the Korean War, the Vietnam War, the Falklands War, the Gulf War and the wars in Afghanistan and Iraq (OEF, OIF in US terminology). The extent that war veterans have embraced PTSD as a diagnostic label and as a collective identity of their mental health status varies by era and country. This variation is related to dominant ideals of masculinity prevailing in the respective cultural and social contexts. Current research literature on PTSD as a diagnosis of war veterans' health symptoms is used here to illuminate this variation.

The first writings about the effects of war on men's mental health portray the experiences of the veterans of World War I (1914-18) (Jones 2006; Mosse 2000; Levy and Sidel 2009; Karner 1995, 2008). As Mosse (2000) has shown, war was regarded as a test of manliness in the nineteenth century. A 'true man' was in control of himself and during World War I the sufferers of 'shell-shock' were perceived to have failed this test. Hence, shell-shock became a metaphor for unmanly behaviour and of an 'enfeebled manhood'.

The impact of World War II (1939–45) covered a whole generation of men. In some countries the 'cult of the fallen soldier', which glorified manliness and national glory, was broken after this war, for example, in Germany (Mosse 1990: 222). In the allied countries, studies of veterans' mental health symptoms suggest that their being welcomed home as heroes, a broad community support for their sacrifices for the nation and for peace, and later support networks of veteran organizations buffered the long-term effects of trauma from that war (Fontana and Rosenheck 1994; see also Hautamäki and Coleman 2001). These studies are mostly based on a rather old cohort of war veterans and their memories and constructed health narratives of their war experiences (e.g. Burnell *et al.* 2010; Hunt 2010).

The study of the mental health of soldiers at war began in a systematic way with the Korean War and its aftermath. The Korean War veterans were not welcomed as heroes to the same extent as World War II veterans or Vietnam War veterans in the US, because the goals of the war were opaque to the general public. The result is that the Korean War veterans have been found to have suffered from mental health symptoms to a greater extent than veterans of World War II and the Vietnam War (Fontana and Rosenheck 1994; Karner 1995, 2008).

The Vietnam War was a long war (1965–75) and its character and cohort of men changed over time. The veterans began upon return to construct their own interpretation of the health effects of traumatic war memories. The emergence of the PTSD diagnosis coincided with the need to handle the post-war trauma symptoms experienced by the Vietnam War veterans and with the rise of the new science of psychiatry in the US. The construction of a new disease category PTSD in the DSM-III in 1980 was the result of a medicalization of war trauma and the new scientific knowledge and disease-focused approach of American psychiatry (Scott 1993).

Two studies based on the narratives of therapists working at the Veterans Administration medical system (Young 1995) and of Vietnam War veterans undergoing therapy (Karner 1995) trace the claims-making of medical legitimacy of the mental ailments from which the veterans suffered. The Vietnam War veterans resisted the label of mental illness, a diagnosis that was connected with weakness and femininity. Instead, PTSD was viewed as a selective and stress-related effect of combat. The veterans presented their symptoms as a situational disorder that had to be seen as an extreme form of masculine behaviour – hypermasculinity – induced under unusual combat conditions. According to their view, PTSD was caused not by a lack of strength but as a result of extreme forms of traditional masculine behaviour (anger, aggression, emotional distance, violence) demanded and triggered under unusual conditions. Young (1995: 208) names this explanatory framework 'the narrative of survival'. The narrative turned the sufferer from an aggressor into the victim of his own aggression.

For these men, the relocation to civilian life also meant a confrontation with changed gender norms because various social movements of the 1960s and 1970s – anti-war, civil rights, and the women's movement – had brought about a new cultural environment and changed views on gender. The war veterans became emblems of a remasculinization of society in the early 1980s by means of cultural icons in the media and Hollywood narrations (Rambo, the Terminator) (Jeffords 1989, 1994). In this changed cultural climate, a medicalization of hypermasculinity became the framework for how the Vietnam War veterans discursively constructed their mental health problems.

The Gulf War Syndrome (GWS), also called Gulf War Illnesses (GWIs), is an example of how the health impact of war became a 'contested illness' (Showalter 1997; Brown *et al.* 2000; Zavestoski *et al.* 2004; Hyams 2005; Kilshaw 2008a, 2008b). After return from active duty, the Gulf War veterans began to experience a cluster of symptoms (e.g. chronic fatigue, irritability, low libido) that came to be known as Gulf War Syndrome (GWS).

The contested nature of the GWS symptoms, because of the shortness of the war (few were in actual combat during the war, in 1990–1), resulted among the American veterans in a resentment of any psychiatric diagnosis of their ailments. Instead the cause of the ailments was presented as organic (i.e. environmental health hazards) and the diagnosis GWS/GWI was viewed as a unique physical rather than a mental condition (Brown *et al.* 2000). The veterans resisted the PTSD diagnosis, especially its psychiatric label, but they later became involved in a negotiation about the meaning of PTSD (Durodie 2006; Kilshaw 2008b: 226). Kilshaw's (2008a:178–9) study of UK Gulf War veterans in 2001–2 showed that the veterans' narratives of GWS focused on loss of masculinity and the failure to live up to the ideal male soldierly body. They interpreted the experienced illnesses as signs of lack of masculinity and as markers of the disorders of women and the old. As Kilshaw (2008a: 184) concludes: 'Their bodies have transformed from the epitome of militarised masculinity to embodying a lack of virility and manliness'. At a later stage UK and American veterans' version of the meaning of PTSD was that it was a secondary effect of the 'real' GWS as an organic and therefore biomedical disease. Although GWS is a contested environmental illness (Brown *et al.* 2000), the claims-making, based on the external character of toxins, relieved veterans from notions of weakness and from failed masculinity as the cause of the ailments (Karner 2008; Kilshaw 2008b: 231).

British studies of the Falkland War and studies of the veterans of the most recent war in Afghanistan and Iraq show that social support from veteran friends was most important in recovery, while avoidance of talking with family about the war experiences was a pattern that delayed recovery (Burnell *et al.* 2006, 2009, 2010). The most recent American figures show gender differences in the mental health diagnoses among OEF and OIF veterans in the US. Female veterans were younger and more likely to be Black and to be diagnosed for depression than were male veterans who were more frequently diagnosed with PTSD and alcohol use disorders. Furthermore, younger men were at higher risk than older men for being diagnosed with PTSD (Maguen *et al.* 2010).

The findings of Finley's study (2011) of the PTSD accounts of American veterans of the wars in Iraq and Afghanistan echo the results of Kilshaw's (2008a) study on the UK Gulf War veterans' narratives of GWS. The symptoms were perceived as weaknesses and unacceptable male behaviour rather than as signs of an illness.

Endorsing and resisting a medicalization of combat-related mental health problems

The veterans' views of their post-war health problems have over the past forty-five years been anchored in contemporary notions of masculinity. A psychiatric diagnosis has tended in most wars to be perceived by male war veterans as a sign of failed or injured masculinity and therefore a psychiatric label has been resisted. A comparison of the Vietnam War veterans' and the Gulf War veterans' negotiations about a diagnosis illustrate the different ways in which masculinity has been medicalized. Vietnam War veterans presented a claim that PTSD was a product of heightened masculinity – that it was not failed and weak masculinity but a 'toxic hypermasculinity' that caused the mental health problems. Similarly, Gulf War veterans negotiated the meaning of GWS to claim that PTSD was not a mental illness and hence lack of masculinity but a secondary side effect of the real organic and biological cause of GWS.

Hence, in both wars there emerged among the veterans a sense of victimization based on a notion of injured masculinity and in public culture the war veterans became emblems for a revival of a strong and traditional masculinity (Jeffords 1989, 1994). The conservative political climate and related Hollywood narrations in the early 1980s and early 1990s supported the war veterans' constructions of a 'hard body' masculinity that also gave a cultural justification for their diagnosis negotiations.

In conclusion, the research on war veterans and their mental health has pointed to the veterans' active participation in the evaluation and treatment of their ailment. Men have not been passive subjects of medicalization but been involved in the definitional process. War veterans have resisted the psychiatric profession's medicalization of their cultural identity as 'true men' and presented alternative claims about the reason for their mental ailments. Veterans' negotiations of diagnosis have been based on their perception that their own notion of masculinity is pathologized and feminized, ultimately leading to a medicalization of their masculinity. The examples about the contestation of the diagnosis of PTSD illuminate the cultural embeddedness of both mental health and masculinity.

Endorsing medicalization: TDS and ED as signs of male aging

The body in science has often depicted the 'body' as the male body but described it as the gender-neutral and 'natural body'. The male body has not only continued to be portrayed as a natural one but during the past two decades science has, in the words of Barbara Marshall (2008: 22), been 'constructing the aging male body as a site of biomedical intervention'. In this endeavour, men's health is linked to a biological or more recently to a hormonal understanding of 'normal' and 'pathological' bodies. Sex hormones have come to define the male body in the same way as was the case with the female hormonal body in the past, as a materialization of the proper hormonal levels because they serve as the chemical messengers of sex (Oudshoorn 1994; Roberts 2007). Any pathologies, according to this biochemical understanding of the body, are related to a deficiency in hormonal level.

The reason for science's newly expressed interest in the male body is the promotion of active sexuality as a marker not only of normal but also of a healthy male aging (Marshall 2008). This intervention represents a new medical view of men's sexual health, which flags androgen deficiency and testosterone deficiency as a broader health problem for aging men (Marshall 2002, 2007, 2008; Baglia 2005). As Fishman (2010) and Watkins (in this volume) have pointed out, this reductionist view departs from the past psychological view of men's impotence. Impotence is no longer located in the realm of men's psyche but since the late 1990s a new biochemical understanding of the male body interprets impotence as a physiological malfunction. While the risks and benefits of hormone replacement therapy for aging women have a long history of critical assessment by women's health advocates and medical researchers, a similar broader critical assessment of testosterone replacement therapy by advocates for men's health seems so far to be relatively invisible.

Hence, andrology has been promoted by the medical profession, for example, urologists, as a field dealing with the new interest in aging men's sexual health. The promotion of testosterone and androgen replacement as a medical treatment for aging men's sexuality is part of the professional claims to present andrology as a new medical specialty that also advances aging men's general health. For example the *Journal of Andrology* has become an important publication channel for evidence-based reviews and recommendations for the new kinds of medical interventions that revitalize aging men's sexual health. Such a view is exemplified in articles published in research and review articles in the *Journal of Andrology* and the *Journal of Men's Health* on the health impact of testosterone deficiency but also on the preventive impact of androgen and testosterone supplementation therapy.

Androgen deficiency is depicted as a new health risk for aging men (see also Watkins's contribution in this volume). As a review article suggests, 'The interest in possible medical intervention to promote healthy aging has been increasing, as the absolute number and the proportion of men over 60 years of age is expected to increase during the next few decades in various countries' (Wald et al. 2006: 126). An article in the *Journal of Men's Health* (Feeley et al. 2009: 173) confirms that 'androgen deficiency is often associated with many pathological states and has adverse effects on men's health'. The adverse effects are loss of muscle strength and impaired sexual functioning, but also a number of chronic diseases such as diabetes and metabolic syndrome and coronary heart disease (e.g. Basaria 2008; Gruenewald and Matsumoto 2003). Medical intervention is promoted in the form of testosterone supplementation because of the 'beneficial role that androgens might have in preventing or ameliorating cardiovascular risk in androgen-deficient men' (Traish et al. 2009b: 490). A number of articles echo this message: 'New clinical information is emerging linking T deficiency to the development of pathology of MetS, diabetes and vascular disease' (Traish et al. 2009a: 18). Another article notes, 'low T could be a predictive marker for those men at high risk of CVD' (Traish et al. 2009b: 477).

In the early days of the medicalization of androgen deficiency among aging men, the major focus was on how to treat erectile dysfunction (ED) and how to restore or enhance sexual performance with Viagra, the brand name of a potency drug that came on the market in 1998. Viagra was not only a concrete drug intervention; it was also a metaphor for a new thinking about the male body (Loe 2001, 2006; Baglia 2005). The metaphor captured male fantasies and cultural images of male sexuality, and this drug has created an enormous illegal drug market via mail order on the internet.

Since the late 2000s the biomedical approach has promoted a new representation of erectile dysfunction (ED): it is a medical marker of prevailing or future chronic diseases among aging men. As one article notes, 'Formerly dismissed as a psychological condition, ED is now known as a treatable disorder and an important risk marker for cardiovascular disease' (Yassin and Saad 2008: 593). For example, a recent review article (Miner 2011) based on studies on ED published during 1998–2009 poses the question: 'Could erectile function serve as a surrogate measure of treatment efficacy of preventive interventions for cardiac disease?' The review provides an affirmative answer: 'ED is an index of subclinical coronary disease and a precursor of cardiovascular (CVS) events' (Miner 2011: 125). The article concludes: 'ED is a potent predictor of all-cause death and the composite of CVS death, MI, stroke, and heart failure in men with CVD' (Miner 2011: 132).

As the above quotations from mainstream men's health journals show, there is a call for a new approach to aging men's health: sexual health is a window to and a messenger of men's general health. For this purpose new agents of medicalization have been introduced. An article about testosterone therapy summarizes the change: 'The recent shift in the management and evaluation of ED, with primary care physicians replacing urologists in the forefront of ED diagnosis and therapy, has been a welcome and timely change' (Yassin and Saad 2008: 600). The article suggests a new stage in the medicalization of men's aging. The first stage was the definition of ED as pathological for aging men and Viagra as the technical solution. The current stage is the establishment of ED as a marker of known chronic diseases among aging men. ED is presented as a screening device and hormonal supplementation as a preventive measure for aging men. In this phase of the medicalization process, it is suggested that the detection and treatment of ED among aging men be turned over to primary care physicians.

In conclusion, the past decade has witnessed the emergence of a sexualized male-gendered body in contrast to the universal and gender-neutral norm that reigned in past medical literature. The aim of this review of the medicalization of TDS among aging men has been to deconstruct the knowledge-making about discursively constituted aging male bodies in scientific discourse. The medicalization of men's health, especially their sexual health, has served as an example in illuminating the emergence of a new representation of the aging male body. The sexed male body has paradoxically received its sexual content by decontexualizing it and drawing on its presocial, biological essence: the hormonal male body needs to be restored to the healthy biologically fixed norm. This image of the hormonal male body has not been resisted among men, as has been the case with PTDS diagnosis among war veterans, but has instead been tacitly endorsed.

A comparison of the processes of medicalization of aging men's health: PTSD and TDS

Medicalization is an analytical framework whereby men's health, masculinity, and aging can be understood and explained. Aging men's health has been used here as a case to illustrate the complex character of medicalization. Aging men's physical and mental symptoms have not only been subjected to new medical labels but men have themselves also been actively involved in resisting certain labels. This chapter has used PTSD and TDS/ED as case studies that illuminate the resistance to and the endorsement of medicalization of aging among men. A comparison of the process and character of medicalization in these two cases points to both differences and similarities.

First, the agents of medicalization differ. In the case of PTDS, war veterans have resisted the medical discourse about their mental symptoms and have negotiated an alternative diagnosis that has freed them from a pathologization of failed masculinity and instead endorsed a diagnosis based on external environmental causes of their symptoms. A medicalization of masculinity has been endorsed by war veterans only if it has pointed to a hypermasculinity induced under perceived extreme external conditions, as in the case of Vietnam War veterans.

In the case of TDS, the agent has been medical specialists (urologists) who were called to restore men's sexual capacity (ED) with a potency drug (Viagra); but, more recently, primary care physicians have been called to screen aging men for ED as a marker for silent or future chronic illnesses like heart disease. The medical focus on sexual health – that is, the detection of ED – has changed from an enhancement procedure to a marker in epidemiological screening and in the prevention of major chronic diseases among aging men.

Second, the claims for medicalization bear some interesting similarities. In both the case of PTSD and TDS, masculinity is defined as a fixed category. In the case of PTSD, masculinity is a fixed cultural script; and in the case of TDS, masculinity is a fixed and static biological and hormonal norm that enables a definition of androgen deficiency. In both cases, the fixed cultural or biological norm not only confirms normality but also produces a definition of a deviation from the norm and a pathologization of that deviation. The deviation is associated with weakness and femininity and in both the cases of PTSD/GWS and TDS with fatigue, loss of libido and impotence. The notions of fatigue associated with GWS were in the veterans' narratives connected with the demasculinizing effects of aging, that is, with 'old people's diseases' and 'old women's diseases' (Kilshaw 2008a: 177).

Third, the medicalization process illustrates the two current theoretical frameworks for understanding the character of medicalization. The case of PTSD illustrates the current phase of medicalization, which a number of sociologists have brought attention to: direct consumer involvement in health issues and the weaker power of the medical profession in the medicalization process. By contrast, the case of TDS exemplifies the process of biomedicalization. This concept, introduced by Clarke and her colleagues (2003, 2010), aims to capture how the interaction of technoscience, biomedical professionals and pharmaceutical corporations produce a discursively constructed hormonal male body and practices related to aging men's sexual health.

The review of the research on PTSD and TDS flags a number of weaknesses in the theorizing on men's health. First, the research on war veterans' mental health constructs the category of 'war veterans' as a gender-neutral category; or, if the gender of the veterans is identified, 'masculinity' is treated as a static trait. This gender representation reproduces the binary gender division as the major social division in society and in this way racial, class and sexual differences are ignored (Jeffords 1989: 179; Schofield 2010: 243). Second, the lack of a vibrant and diverse theoretical knowledge production about men's health results in an unchallenged position for the biomedical discourse on men's health, as exemplified in the case of TDS and ED as signs of male aging. Finally, sociological research on men's health has been characterized by a theoretical diffuseness compared to early theorizing on women's health, which was characterized by different and distinct theoretical approaches (Fee 1977). The valorization of a cultural explanations of men's health and health behaviour (e.g. Courtenay 2000; O'Brien *et al.* 2005) has given men's health advocates few analytical tools other than a cultural (often a sex-role theory) approach to the health of aging men. In theorizing on men's health, new inroads have recently flagged the importance of considering class, race and ethnicity in examining and understanding men's health (e.g. Lohan 2007; Evans *et al.* 2011; Dolan 2011).

References

Abraham, J. (2010) 'Pharmaceuticalization of society in context: Theoretical, empirical and health dimensions', *Sociology*, 44: 603–22.
Baglia, J. (2005) *The Viagra Adventure: Masculinity, Media, and the Performance of Sexual Health*, New York: Peter Lang.
Basaria, S. (2008) 'Androgen deprivation therapy, insulin resistance, and cardiovascular mortality: An inconvenient truth', *Journal of Andrology*, 29: 534–9.
Bracken, P. J. (2001) 'Post-modernity and post-traumatic stress disorder', *Social Science and Medicine*, 53: 733–43.
Broom, A., and Tovey, P. (eds) (2010) *Men's Health: Body, Identity and Social Context*, Chichester: John Wiley-Blackwell.
Brown, P., Zavestoksi, S., McCormick, S., Linder, M., Mandelbaum, J., and Luebke, T. (2000) 'A gulf of difference: Disputes over Gulf War-related illnesses', *Journal of Health and Social Behavior*, 42: 235–57.
Burnell, K. J., Coleman, P. G., and Hunt, N. (2006) 'Falklands War veterans' perceptions of social support and the reconciliation of traumatic memories', *Aging and Mental Health*, 10: 282–9.
Burnell, K. J., Hunt, N., and Coleman, P. G. (2009) 'Developing a model of narrative analysis to investigate the role of social support in coping with traumatic war memories', *Narrative Inquiry*, 19: 91–105.
Burnell, K. J., Coleman, P. G., and Hunt, N. (2010) 'Coping with traumatic memories: Second World War veterans' experiences of social support in relation to the narrative coherence of war memories', *Ageing and Society*, 30: 57–78.
Busfield, J. (1996) *Men, Women and Madness: Understanding Gender and Mental Disorder*, London: Macmillan Press.
Chesler, P. (1989) *Women and Madness*, New York: Harcourt Brace Jovanovich (orig. 1972).
Clarke, A. E., Shim, J. K., Mamo, L., Fosket, J. R., and Fishman, J. R. (2003) 'Biomedicalization: Technoscientific transformations of health, illness, and U.S. biomedicine', *American Sociological Review*, 68: 161–94.
Clarke, A. E., Mamo, L., Fosket, J. R., Fishman, J. R., and Shim, J. K. (eds) (2010) *Biomedicalization: Technoscience, Health, and Illness in the US*, Durham, NC: Duke University Press.

Connell, R.W., and Messerschmidt, J. W. (2005) 'Hegemonic masculinity: Rethinking the concept', *Gender and Society*, 19: 829–59.
Conrad, P. (2005) 'The shifting engines of medicalization', *Journal of Health and Social Behavior*, 46: 3–14.
Conrad, P. (2007) *The Medicalization of Society: On the Transformation of Human Conditions into Treatable Disorders*, Baltimore, MD: Johns Hopkins University Press.
Courtenay, W. (2000) 'Constructions of masculinity and their influence on men's well-being: A theory of gender and health', *Social Science and Medicine*, 50: 1385–1401.
Dolan, A. (2011) '"You can't ask for a Dubonnet and lemonade!": Working class masculinity and men's health practices', *Sociology of Health and Illness*, 33: 586–601.
Durodie, B. (2006) 'Risk and the social construction of "Gulf War Syndrome"', *Philosophical Transactions of the Royal Society*, 361: 689–95.
Evans, J., Frank, B., Oliffe, J. L., and Gregory, D. (2011) 'Health, illness, men and masculinities (HIMM): A theoretical framework for understanding men and their health', *Journal of Men's Health*, 8: 7–11.
Fee, E. (1977) 'Women and health care: A comparison of theories', in V. Navarro (ed.), *Health and Medical Care in the USA: A Critical Analysis*, Farmingdale, NY: Baywood Publishing.
Feeley, R. J., Saad, F., Guay, A., and Traish, A.M. (2009) 'Testosterone in men's health: A new role for an old hormone', *Journal of Men's Health*, 6: 169–76.
Finley, E. P. (2011) *Fields of Combat: Understanding PTSD among Veterans of Iraq and Afghanistan*, Ithaca, NY: Cornell University Press.
Fishman, J. R. (2010) 'The making of Viagra: The biomedicalization of sexual dysfunction', in A. E. Clarke, L. Mamo, J. R. Fosket, J. R. Fishman, and J. K. Shim (eds), *Biomedicalization: Technoscience, Health, and Illness in the US*, Durham, NC: Duke University Press.
Fontana, A., and Rosenheck, R. (1994) 'Traumatic war stressors and psychiatric symptoms among World War II, Korean, and Vietnam War veterans', *Psychology and Aging*, 9: 27–33.
Fox, N. J., and Ward, K. J. (2008) 'Pharma in the bedroom ... and the kitchen ... The pharmaceuticalisation of daily life', *Sociology of Health and Illness*, 30: 856–68.
Gruenewald, D. A., and Matsumoto, A. M. (2003) 'Testosterone supplementation therapy for older men: Potential benefits and risks', *Journal of American Geriatrics*, 51: 101–15.
Hautamäki, A., and Coleman, P. G. (2001) 'Explanation for low prevalence of PTSD among older Finnish war veterans: Social solidarity and continued significance given to wartime sufferings', *Aging and Mental Health*, 5: 165–74.
Hunt, N. C. (2010) *Memory, War and Trauma*, Cambridge: Cambridge University Press.
Hutchings, K. (2008) 'Making sense of masculinity and war', *Men and Masculinities*, 10: 389–404.
Hyams, K. C. (2005) 'Adding to our comprehension of Gulf War health questions', *International Journal of Epidemiology*, 34: 808–9.
Jeffords, S. (1989) *The Remasculinization of America: Gender and the Vietnam War*, Bloomington, IN: Indiana University Press.
Jeffords, S. (1994) *Hard Bodies: Hollywood Masculinity in the Reagan Era*, New Brunswick, NJ: Rutgers University Press.

Jones, E. (2006) 'Historical approaches to post-combat disorders', *Philosophical Transactions of the Royal Society*, 361: 533–42.
Karner, T. X. (1995) 'Medicalizing masculinity: Post traumatic stress disorder in Vietnam veterans', *Masculinities*, 3: 23–65.
Karner, T. X. (2008) 'Post-traumatic stress disorder and older men: If only time healed all wounds', *Generations*, 32: 82–7.
Kempner, J. (2006) 'Uncovering man in medicine: Lessons learned from a case study of cluster headache', *Gender and Society*, 20: 632–56.
Kilshaw, S. (2008a) *Impotent Warriors: Gulf War Syndrome, Vulnerability and Masculinity*, New York: Berghahn Books.
Kilshaw, S. (2008b) 'Gulf War Syndrome: A reaction to psychiatry's invasion of the military?', *Culture, Medicine and Psychiatry*, 32: 219–37.
Levy, B. S., and Sidel, V. W. (2009) 'Health effects of combat: A life course perspective', *Annual Review of Public Health*, 30: 123–36.
Loe, M. (2001) 'Fixing broken masculinity: Viagra as a technology for the production of gender and sexuality', *Sexuality and Culture*, 5: 97–125.
Loe, M. (2006) '"The Viagra blues": Embracing or resisting the Viagra body', in D. Rosenfeld and C. A. Faircloth (eds), *Medicalized Masculinities*, Philadelphia, PA: Temple University Press.
Lohan, M. (2007) 'How might we understand men's health better? Integrating explanations from critical studies on men and inequalities in health', *Social Science and Medicine*, 65: 493–504.
Lunbeck, E. (1998) 'American psychiatrists and the modern man, 1900 to 1920', *Men and Masculinities*, 1: 58–86.
Lupton, D. (1997) 'Foucault and the medicalization critique', in A. Petersen and R. Bunton (eds), *Foucault: Health and Medicine*, London: Routledge.
Maguen, S., Ren, L. Bosch, J. O., Marmar, C. R., and Seal, K. H. (2010) 'Gender differences in mental health diagnoses among Iraq and Afghanistan veterans enrolled in Veterans Affairs health care', *American Journal of Public Health*, 100: 2450–6.
Marshall, B. L. (2002) '"Hard science": Gendered constructions of sexual dysfunction in the "Viagra age"', *Sexualities*, 5: 131–58.
Marshall, B. L. (2007) 'Climacteric redux? (Re)medicalizing the male menopause', *Men and Masculinities*, 9: 509–29.
Marshall, B. L. (2008) 'Older men and sexual health: Post-Viagra views of changes in function', *Generations*, 32: 21–7.
Miner, M. M. (2011) 'Erectile dysfunction: A harbinger or consequence. Does its detection lead to a window of curability?', *Journal of Andrology*, 32: 125–34.
Mosse, G. L. (1990) *Fallen Soldiers: Reshaping the Memory of the World Wars*, Oxford: Oxford University Press.
Mosse, G. L. (2000) 'Shell-shock as a social disease', *Journal of Contemporary History*, 35: 101–8.
O'Brien, R., Hunt, K., and Hart, G. (2005) '"It's caveman stuff, but that is to certain extent how guys still operate": Men's accounts of masculinity and help seeking', *Social Science and Medicine*, 61: 503–16.
Oliffe, J (2006) 'Embodied masculinity and androgen deprivation therapy', *Sociology of Health and Illness*, 28: 410–32.
Oudshoorn, N. (1994) *Beyond the Natural Body: Archeology of Sex Hormones*, London: Routledge.

Riessman, C. K. (1983) 'Women and medicalization: A new perspective', *Social Policy* (summer): 3–19.
Riska, E. (2003) 'Gendering the medicalization thesis', *Advances in Gender Research*, 7: 59–87.
Roberts, C. (2007) *Messengers of Sex: Hormones, Biomedicine and Feminism*, Cambridge: Cambridge University Press.
Rosenfeld, D., and Faircloth, C. (eds) (2006) *Medicalized Masculinities*, Philadephia, PA: Temple University Press.
Sabo, D., and Gordon, F. (eds) (1995) *Men's Health and Illness: Gender, Power and the Body*, London: Sage.
Schofield, T. (2010) 'Men's health and well-being', in E. Kuhlmann and E. Annandale (eds), *Handbook of Gender and Healthcare*, Basingstoke: Palgrave.
Scott, W. J. (1993) *The Politics of Readjustment: Vietnam Veterans since the War*, New York: Aldine de Gruyter.
Showalter, E. (1997) *Hystories: Hysterical Epidemics and Modern Media*, New York: Columbia University Press.
Traish, A. M., Guay, A., Feeley, R., and Saad, F. (2009a) 'The dark side of testosterone deficiency: I. metabolic syndrome and erectile dysfunction', *Journal of Andrology*, 30: 10–22.
Traish, A. M., Saad, F., Feeley, R. J., and Guay, A. (2009b) 'The dark side of testosterone deficiency: III. cardiovascular disease', *Journal of Andrology*, 30: 477–94.
Wald, M., Meacham, R. B., Ross, L. S., and Niederberger, C. S. (2006) 'Testosterone replacement therapy for older men', *Journal of Andrology*, 27: 126–32.
Williams, S. J., Martin, P., and Gabe, J. (2011) 'The pharmaceuticalisation of society? A framework for analysis', *Sociology of Health and Illness*, 33: 710–25.
Yassin, A. A., and Saad, F. (2008) 'Testosterone and erectile dysfunction', *Journal of Andrology*, 29: 593–604.
Young, A. (1995) *The Harmony of Illusions: Inventing Post-traumatic Disorder*, Princeton, NJ: Princeton University Press.
Zavestoski, S., Brown, P., McCormick, S., Mayer, B., D'Ottavi, M., and Lucove, J. C. (2004) 'Patient activism and the struggle for diagnosis: Gulf War illnesses and other medically unexplained physical symptoms in the US', *Social Science and Medicine*, 58: 161–75.
Zola, I. K. (1972) 'Medicine as an institution of social control', *Sociological Review*, 20: 487–504.

5 The vicissitudes of 'healthy aging'

The experiences of older migrant men in a rural Australian community

Susan Feldman, Alan Petersen and Harriet Radermacher

This chapter investigates the experiences of older men from culturally and linguistically diverse (CALD) backgrounds and in doing so seeks to challenge the dominant biomedical perspective on aging. Within biomedicine, aging tends to be seen as a process of inexorable decline, decay and dependency, with the focus of many interventions being on correcting biophysical 'defects' or 'malfunctioning', to enable its 'successful' fulfilment ('healthy aging'). In the case of aging males, these assumptions can be seen clearly in the strong focus on 'sexual dysfunction' and on correcting impotence through the use of various techniques and technologies, such as Viagra, to restore an idealized 'normal, healthy' masculine sexuality (see e.g. Fishman 2010). A whole subfield of biomedicine and pharmaceutical industry has emerged as a consequence (Loe 2004). Drawing on the findings from a qualitative study of how older CALD men living in a rural community perceive and make sense of their own health and well-being, we question this biomedical conception of healthy male aging. This study was undertaken in rural Australia (Victoria) from 2009 to 2011 and involves men from Italian, Macedonian, Turkish and Albanian backgrounds. Service providers and community leaders also contributed their views and thus enabled us to identify the challenges they face in addressing the health needs of this group of men. The study underlines the importance of considering the complex and interconnecting experiences of migration, gender, family and personal identity in understanding the men's lives. In particular, it indicates the need for supportive interventions that go beyond a focus on narrowly defined concepts of 'health' to pay cognizance to the various influences of men's experiences.

Why worry about older CALD men in rural Australia?

The Australian *National Men's Health Policy* highlighted the neglected needs of a number of groups including men in rural communities (Department of Health and Ageing 2008). Men who live in rural communities are subject to a number of disadvantages, especially if they are old and from a CALD background. Over a quarter of Australia's population was born overseas (Australian Bureau of Statistics 2011). Compared to those who live in urban areas, people are more likely to be vulnerable to a range of diseases and premature death and to engage in behaviours that put their health at risk. They also have a lower level of health literacy than their urban counterparts (Australian Institute of Health and Welfare 2010), and have less access to health and support services than their metropolitan counterparts. For rural men, risk factors may include social isolation, high unemployment, economic hardship and population decline and poor access to mental health services (Department of Health and Ageing 2008).

Many older rural men are employed, or have been employed before retirement, in the physically demanding agricultural industry. This work often requires them to deal with the stress of working in socially isolated conditions, extreme environmental changes such as drought and fire, and under the constant threat of unemployment. Older men who have played the 'bread-winner' role are likely to resist retiring from the workforce, despite changes to their physical and mental capacity, or may experience a severe disruption to their identity upon retirement since they are likely to lose their connections to significant networks (Granville and Evandrou 2010). The struggle to cope with life changes has been reported as contributing to high levels of stress, anxiety and increasing suicide rates in older men (Jensen *et al.* 2010). Older people who have experienced an accumulation of stressful events and daily hassles are at greater risk of poor mental health (Kraaij *et al.* 2002); and the coping strategies commonly used by older men in stressful situations lead to poor psychological adjustment (Jensen *et al.* 2010; Addis and Mahalik 2003). Mental health is at further risk due to older rural men being less likely to seek professional assistance for health disorders (Council on the Ageing 2008).

While a growing body of evidence highlights the particular problems faced by men in rural communities (e.g. Australian Institute of Health and Welfare 2010), there has been scant reference to older men, let alone those from CALD communities. In government policy and practice, this is an invisible, marginalized group, whose particular needs have been largely neglected. Men from CALD backgrounds may encounter specific barriers to maintaining their mental health and well-being, which include: lack of English language skills; stigma associated with seeking support; lack of culturally appropriate information about available services; and inequitable access to community aged care services (Fuller *et al.* 2000; Kiropoulos *et al.* 2005; Radermacher *et al.* 2009). Older men, especially those from a non-dominant ethnic community, are likely to experience a threat to their identity and sense of well-being as they age, since they tend to encounter greater difficulty in maintaining cultural and social connections to their communities (Constant *et al.* 2006). Furthermore, the needs of CALD groups are more likely to be neglected in rural locations (Pugh *et al.* 2007). There is an increasing demand for more effective and culturally appropriate management of health problems via coordinated and integrated primary care services, particularly in rural areas (Bambling *et al.* 2007; Fuller *et al.* 2000; Sweeney and Kisely 2003).

While this chapter focuses on the experiences of men from four different CALD groups, we acknowledge the importance of not treating older men as a homogeneous group with common experiences, which may lead to incorrect assumptions and the stereotyping of particular groups. As with the Anglo-Australian community, there is much diversity and heterogeneity within CALD communities and individuals will differ in any number of ways (e.g. values, religion, practices, etc.). Furthermore, the study on which this chapter is based was not comparative; rather it sought to examine the range and nature of the participants' experiences.

This chapter addresses four intersecting elements namely age, ethnicity, gender and rural location. It is only by examining all four elements in combination that our understanding about the complex nature of growing old as a CALD man in rural Australia can be enhanced.

Our study

Semi-structured individual and group interviews were conducted with 13 individuals representing health and service organizations and ethnic community leaders; 26 older CALD men (from Albanian, Turkish, Italian and Macedonian backgrounds); and four older women from Albanian and Italian backgrounds. The CALD men had an average age of 66 (ranging from 39 to 85 years); the majority of whom were married ($n=24$), and had children. While this study sought the opinions of men over 60, a number of younger men (e.g. the Turkish and Albanian imams), who were integral to the recruitment of the older men, also took part. Most lacked post-school qualifications. They had a range of health conditions (including heart disease, diabetes, musculoskeletal conditions, high blood pressure and Parkinson's disease), and their current/previous occupations included orchardists, labourers and farmers. All interviews took place in local, community venues. To ensure the anonymity of participants, we have not identified the particular location in which the study was undertaken. Bilingual interpreters were used as required. Quotes are presented verbatim from a range of individual participants, without corrections to the English, and if they are the words of the interpreter it is noted in the text.

Guiding concepts

The absence of theory is a common criticism of the gerontological field and, where theory has been applied, it has rarely explained the lives of older immigrants (McDonald 2011). As McDonald (2011: 1192) argues, 'at best' theories have provided 'several different lenses through which to examine immigration and its effects on the physical, social and psychological aspects of aging', but often these theories have not been explicitly applied. Indeed it may be pertinent to question whether these theories of aging are inclusive of and have taken into account the perspectives of older migrants. Torres (2004) asserts that international migrants have remained on the periphery of theory development within social gerontology, which she cautions is an oversight given the hybridity that is so characteristic of the international migrant experience and the wealth of insight their experience can offer. Notions of what it means to experience 'healthy aging' are 'contextually determined' and therefore may be characterised by change and fluidity (Torres 2004).

In developing our perspective, we have found the life-course approach invaluable, in offering a structure or 'scaffold' through which to accommodate and promote interdisciplinary theory building (McDonald 2011). Bengston *et al.* (2005) identified five principles that define the life-course perspective: (1) lives are interconnected; (2) social and historical context shape individual lives; (3) transitions and their timing are influenced by the social contexts in which individuals make choices; (4) individuals are active agents in the construction of their lives; and (5) relationships, events and behaviours of earlier life stages have consequences for later life relationships, statuses and well-being. In addition, Atchley's theories of adaptation (1998) and continuity (1989, 1999) offer insights into how adults – in this case older CALD men – continuously learn from their lifetime experiences, and progressively develop in the direction determined by their intentional, conscious and active preferences. Of particular relevance to this study is Atchley's continuity theory which is concerned with understanding how individuals avoid or minimize the effects of role loss by maintaining their long-standing activities or structures (Atchley 1998: 21). Together these principles provide a useful framework from which to understand the experiences of the men in this study.

The concept of healthy aging

As noted, the field of aging studies has been dominated by the biomedical perspective that sees the process of aging as involving illness, decay, decline and growing dependency. Consequently, aging has tended to be viewed as a deficit and the problems experienced by older people have been treated as a form of pathology. It is of course a fallacy to presume that all older people are ill, that old age is synonymous with failing health, mental decline and physical deterioration. We do not of course argue that there are no medical implications of growing old and longevity, but would advocate the importance of distinguishing between changes that tend to accompany the process of biological aging and those that are linked to the disease process.

Chronological age has been used by many scholars as a surrogate measure of 'being old' because chronological age defines membership in a cohort group and adds a historical perspective to an individual's experiences across the life course. This is despite there being little agreement about at what point a person can be described as being old (Rowland 1991). Of course, chronological age does have a place when thinking about retirement, service planning and policy issues; however we argue that chronological age is often used inappropriately to capture people's experiences at different stages of life. Sociologists have drawn attention to the social construction of old age, with many noting the rapid changes in definitions of aging and 'the aged' (e.g. Faircloth 2003; Gilleard and Higgs 2005; Vincent 2003, 2008).

Health has been defined as 'a state of complete physical, mental and social well-being and not merely the absence of disease or infirmity' (World Health Organization 1952: 100). While useful, this definition we acknowledge is not without limitations. It has been extensively critiqued, including on the basis that the word 'complete' makes it unlikely that anyone would attain optimum health for any length of time and that the above phrase appears to describe happiness rather than health (see e.g. Saracci 1997; World Health Organization 2011). The concept of 'healthy aging' extends the WHO's perspective, and provides a way to look at some important dimensions of 'aging well'. Recent trends have seen researchers adopt a more multidisciplinary, psychosocial approach to understanding the complex process of growing older. Researchers are posing new questions about quality of life, as experienced and reported by older people themselves (e.g. relationships, housing, transport, economic circumstances). Healthy, or 'successful', aging has been conceptualized as comprising three hierarchical components: low risk of disease and disability, high physical and mental functioning, and active engagement with life (Rowe and Kahn 1998). Subsequent definitions have emphasized the additional importance of spirituality (Crowther *et al.* 2002; McCann Mortimer *et al.* 2008; Tohit *et al.* 2012), particularly when researchers have included the perspectives of people outside of traditional White and Western parameters. Healthy aging is in active opposition to 'ageism' – a perspective that associates older age with physical and mental decline and portrays older people as obnoxious complainers, 'bed blockers' in public hospitals and a burden to society (Angus and Reeve 2006; Larkin 2001). Moreover, healthy aging is based on the notions that the individual and the environment are interactive, and that positive behavioural outcomes are a direct result of the adaptations and negotiations that take place within this context (Baltes 1996; Baltes and Smith 1999; Vaillant 2002; Vaillant and Mukamal 2001).

Largely due to being dominated by the biomedical perspective, the field of aging studies has until recent years been oblivious to the influence of factors such as gender, ethnicity, migration experience and place of residence. With the increasing attention to a more holistic view of aging, we welcome a greater exploration of how such factors shape people's experiences.

A gendered approach

It is important to note that, in social terms, gender does make a difference in the way life is experienced. While growing older is a process that affects all human beings, we contend that a gendered analysis of the lives of older men and women will provide a better understanding about the systematic inequalities that exist between them across the life course. As the feminist literature and literature on men and masculinity emphasizes, gender is an enactment; it is accomplished through routine social interactions (West and Zimmerman 1987). Dominant masculine ideals that emphasize power, control and stoicism shape the behaviours of men (including their risk and help-seeking behaviours) to varying degrees, influenced by factors including age, ethnicity and place of residence (Galdas 2009). Masculinity is enacted differently in different ethnic minority communities (e.g. Archer 2003; Courtenay 2000; Petersen 1998). Adopting a 'gender lens' in any exploration of the lives of older people enables an examination of the social and structural factors that shed light on the aging experience – consideration of gender being more important than chronological age (Arber *et al.* 2003; Arber and Ginn 1995). To include women and men of different ethnic and socio-economic backgrounds in any analysis of growing older is not only a political act, but good science because it is basic to any understanding of how life is experienced by people and of particular relevance to our study, involving older men from diverse ethnic backgrounds who have different cultural traditions and values.

The focus on gender in aging can be viewed as an appropriate response to a demographic imperative and works against ageist stereotyping of older people who are often viewed as a homogeneous group. This has been noted as a damaging perspective that overlooks the variation and differentiation in the experiences of aging for both women and men (Angus and Reeve 2006). A gendered approach allows for a multi-layered view of the aging experience and one that has implications for better understanding social structures, constraints and cultural values beyond the control of individuals (Calasanti and Slevin 2006).

One way in which to further our understanding about the significance of gender and aging is to examine how men's sense of identity and autonomy in later life is maintained. Men have been described as 'in their prime' between the ages of 45 and 60, dominant in every sphere of society; academia, business, politics and religion (Thompson 1994) and, for a small minority, this power is little diminished even in very old age. Nevertheless, for the majority of men, advancing years heralds removal from 'centre stage' in order to make room for the upcoming 'Young Turks' (Arber *et al.* 2003: 5). As the men in our study alluded to, they are reluctantly resigned to the relinquishing of their role as head of the family and main provider of economic security for their families. As they grow older and their responsibilities diminish, they face a challenge to their identity as prime bread-winner or head of the family, which was established many years earlier, as newly arrived migrants. In face of these changes questions arise about who they are and what they will become as they face changing roles and the aging process.

Migration

Where migrants come from is perhaps less significant than the fact they have a life course characterized by disruption and discontinuity (Torres 2004). This is interesting in light of assumptions that most social gerontologists make about continuity being crucial for 'healthy aging'. The act of migrating invites a 'hybridity' of experience, where migrants are exposed to different cultural attitudes and values that may challenge and contradict their pre-existing beliefs and lead them to question the way they think and live their lives (Torres 2004). This may be unsettling, stressful or, alternatively, a source of strength and a potential resource (Torres 2004). By being forced to renegotiate the world around them, migrants may develop more effective coping strategies, leading to increased self-efficacy and resilience. Hence it may be important to think about the migration experience not only in terms of losses and difficulties, but also with regard to the immense and numerous possibilities that it may bring.

Men in all the groups reinforced the important role of their home country's traditions and culture, and emphasized that it was integral to their identity and well-being. The men talked about the expectation that each generation must provide for the next. This was closely associated to the role they played in their families, as boss of their own home, and of being respected.

Cultural identity

The CALD communities in this study appeared to vary in relation to how much they assimilated with the mainstream Anglo-Australian community, the extent of assimilation being determined by numerous factors including the length of time since migration and English-language proficiency. Regardless of how 'Australianized' migrants perceived themselves to be, their ethnic and cultural background and traditions remained fundamental to their identities, as the following Italian man explained:

> I have no problem to integrate with the Australian community but my blood is Italian blood running around ... I came here at 15 years of age and I've been naturalized since about 17 with my parents, but deep inside I feel Italian.
>
> (Italian male)

These men also appeared to enjoy investing time in maintaining their cultural traditions, by taking part in traditional activities:

> I've been in Australia 72 years now and what I see, what I see is that at our age now, we try to keep the tradition, making wine, making grappa, making salame, you know ... and tell all about the past.
>
> (Italian male)

Spending time with other members from the same ethnic community was a way of life and something that these men did not seem to question. Not only did this appear to maintain their links with their country of origin and traditions, and bolster their own identities, but made them 'feel better'. This comment was made by an Italian who, despite acknowledging that the Italians were well integrated within the broader community, still felt that he was treated as 'non-Aussie'. This was a sentiment that seemed to be supported by a comment from the discussion in the Turkish group, 'Once they are connected with the community and the children they are more happy, they are a lot happier' (Turkish interpreter).

The extent to which the men felt that they could connect to their communities and the land they had left behind was particularly significant for the Turkish group. Of all the groups, it was the Turks who had been in Australia the least amount of time, appearing more isolated from the mainstream community particularly on account of being less proficient in English. They spoke of a longing for home, and described the stark contrast between the life they left behind and the one they were currently living. They talked about how living in rural Australia, with its big, empty, quiet streets, was a world away from the hustle and bustle of street life back in Turkey. They also talked about the potential negative implications of not having access to a constant source of social activity and networks:

> Our culture, we talk too much with the friends, and we are living too close with someone else's, but if you stay alive, if you couldn't visit someone or someone couldn't visit, then psychological problem.
>
> (Turkish male)

Ties with the home country appear to remain strong within the Italian and Turkish groups in particular. With improvements in communication and transportation systems these ties have been maintained, something that was previously more difficult (Torres 2004). The men placed significant importance upon returning to one's home country to connect with people and their 'old' way of life.

However, a commonly reported phenomenon in the literature is that of getting stuck in a time warp; that is, maintaining their original beliefs and cultural practices. Not living in their countries of origin means that they have not moved with the times and their current thinking can become outdated. This is well illustrated by the following comment from an Italian man:

> But our tradition, I went back [to Italy] after 48 years and my aunty in Italy, now she passed away 5 years ago, well, when she heard me speaking, I was speaking exactly the same dialect when I left Italy and to her, I was a magnific [magnificent] thing she said, because she said, today the youngest of today they [makes a sound] you can't hear, you can't understand them anymore. And it's true.
>
> (Italian male)

The migrant experience is inextricably entwined with coming to Australia with little and earning money to build a better life. Possibly for this reason, financial issues were of common concern to the men. This was particularly the case with the Macedonian men, who talked about the high costs of doctors, the increasing cost of running farms and now having to pay for water and their lack of eligibility for the pension (due to having big assets, related to owning land). In their view, they had worked hard, paid taxes and it was time that the government supported them and gave something back. As one observed:

> they came to this country, it was his cousin that brought him here and he stayed here because he wanted to achieve something to make something for himself, but again the government instead of giving them something they're taking from them.
>
> (Macedonian male)

The sense of entitlement and feeling 'hard done by' seemed to be exacerbated by the perception that new migrants coming to Australia do not work and get government benefits:

> Why I shouldn't be? 73 years now. Pay tax and you have to pay the doctor. Other people coming here, they don't work, they get money and they don't pay the doctor.
>
> (Macedonian male)

The role of family

Over the past 100 years the world has witnessed an evolution in the configuration of the modern family, particularly with regards to the complex relationship between 'economic, social and cultural developments and changes in families and households' (Reiger 2005: 44). Within the context of our discussion about the health and well-being of older CALD men we consider 'the ways in which families are shaped by society – by place, time and culture' (Reiger 2005: 43). Families are changing, subject to external and societal forces reflecting changing attitudes, function and values, especially in relation to the place of older family members (Feldman and Seedsman 2005: 194). The men in this study told us that family had always been extremely significant to them. Now that they are aging with diminishing family responsibilities some are openly questioning their future roles within their extended multi-generational family, while at the same time continuing to place great significance on family relationships and cohesion.

Within their discussions around family roles and responsibilities, men also talked specifically about how their wives had provided constant emotional, physical and practical support throughout their marriage. They said women had worked alongside them on their farms, raising children and taking care of the household. An Albanian man described his relationship with his wife as being 'blended into each other'. Other men also felt supported by their wives, noting that in more recent years they had encouraged them to think about their health by cooking them more healthy meals. One Italian man jokingly referred to every man's need for a 'Maria' (i.e. a woman to provide love and support), and this reflected the sentiments expressed by an Italian community leader: 'Normally their [older Italian man's] wife does everything for them you know, it's not like the Aussie wife.' Comparisons such as this were often made with the mainstream Anglo-Australian population. Many participants, for example, were of the opinion that the family unit and the bonds between family members were stronger than those within the mainstream population, as illustrated by this exchange between the interviewer and an Albanian woman:

> But see being ethnic, we're a different breed. Can I say that?
> Q: Yeah, you can. Of course you can. And tell me what different breed means?
> I don't know, we're more family orientated.
> Q: Yeah, you think so?
> Very much so.

The importance of family was connected to the seemingly high expectations that participants had about their children, particularly their achievements and their own relationships with them. In their opinion, children should provide care and support to their aging parents. This attitude is perhaps not surprising when one considers that many of these men migrated to Australia in their youth, seeking a better life not only for themselves but for their children. They saw Australia as providing both them and their children with better educational and employment opportunities. These expectations were also linked to the importance of maintaining a sense of family pride and honour, as expressed by an Italian interpreter, and was confirmed by an older Italian participant and his wife:

> I think with the Italians and all the Europeans too, you want to feel as though you're a good standing in the community, your job gives you honour, your house gives you honour, your family gives you honour. If somebody in the family is not cooperating with the family he gives kind of a black picture, so they don't like that ... And of course when they want to have their friends looking at them they want them to think, 'oh they're lucky people, everything is going well for them'.
>
> (Italian interpreter)

There was, however, a sense of ambivalence about the role of children in the older men's lives. The men acknowledged that times are changing, that children are busy and have their own lives and families. There was also an understanding that their children are more 'Australianized', and they don't necessarily want to take on the family business, marry within the community and live in the same town.

> What asset? Who wants the land? Who wants the ground? Who wants to work? I've got one boy ... any time I let him go. What future in land?
> Q: *Where he wants to go?*
> Oh, he marry.
> Q: *He wants to leave [name of regional town]. Does he?*
> He wants to leave the orchard.
> Q: *To get off the orchard?*
> Too many worries. Well, there is no money and the water is too much.
> (Macedonian male)

In addition, the men were clear that they did not want to be an additional burden on their kids. However, there was still a longing for a family that was close and maintained ongoing contact and communication:

> Biggest problem is when the children grow up; we would like to still interact with them. Once that happens, when they don't interact with us, that's when they feel so sad. Yeah, unhappy.
> (Turkish interpreter)

The changes in these older migrant men's attitudes towards familial obligations can possibly be explained by the acceptance that their children have grown up in a society that equates successful aging with autonomy, independence and self-determination (Torres 2004). This is in stark contrast to many migrants' pre-existing cultural beliefs that aging well is synonymous with dependence upon the younger generation to take care of them as they grow older. Torres refers to the notion of 'in-between' cultures to try to explain what happens when migrants try and negotiate combining the cultural beliefs and traditions that they have grown up with and bring with them, with those of their new host nation.

A life-course perspective

The interaction between gender and migration can produce very different life courses for men and women (Maynard *et al.* 2008). Because of the strong significance of change in the lives of the men in this study, a life-course perspective is a useful tool to think about concepts such as healthy aging, adaptation, continuity, migration, gender and identity.

These men's lives are interwoven with those of their families foremost, as well as with those from their country of origin. Their lives, to some extent, have been determined by their geographic location and the changing economic climate and this has subsequently had an impact on their relationships with others. The changes in the agricultural industry (for example, increasing water prices, regulations, drought), coupled with children growing up in Australia where traditional Australian cultural values emphasize autonomy and education, have resulted in children deciding not to take on family businesses, and moving to bigger towns away from the family.

Clearly, coming from impoverished and often restrictive Communist regimes has shaped and continues to shape the way in which some of the men have chosen to live their lives in Australia – with an emphasis on working hard and gaining financial security. These men have been active agents in their own lives, but possibly their life choices (or their perceptions of the opportunities) have been fairly narrow and limited to paid employment and orientated to family. For the Albanian and Turkish men, their Muslim faith has been a solid structure upon which they have made choices about how they have led their lives. For Italian men, Catholicism has played a similar role.

As we previously outlined, ideas related to how an individual navigates the course of their life through the necessary changes and adjustments can provide a comprehensive understanding about the quality of the life and the associated priorities for people as they age. In this case the majority of men in our study had migrated to Australia as young boys who had left their homeland in search of a better life. As non-English-speaking migrants they were willing to work hard to achieve a better quality of life and in particular secure their economic future. Despite their young age, most of the men arrived in Australia with established patterns of hard physical work and traditional beliefs firmly intact, particularly those in relation to the male role as bread-winner and provider for the family. As a consequence, work had played a vital role over the following decades in not only shaping the economic direction of the course of their lives, but also in relation to their male identities. Of particular significance to the men was the part that their work had played in confirming their identities as head of the family and associated ongoing responsibilities that included their extended family networks. Over the ensuing years these men had developed and maintained an exceptionally strong sense of identity and belonging to their communities and country of origin, and strong bonds with their families.

Consequently, for these men, maintaining a sense of purpose, place and identity across the life course remained bound up with their long established patterns of work, family and community responsibilities. Despite their increasing age and changing physical capacity some men expressed a desire to continue to be seen as contributing members of their family through their involvement in physical work related to the agricultural industry. As one Macedonian man said: 'What am I supposed to do if I stop working? And it's not good to stop working, because we're used to working.' There was evidence to suggest that the men were 'compensating' for a decline in their physical functioning. For example, while the majority of the Macedonian men still seemed to be working long hours on their family orchards, the nature of their contributions were changing, as an interpreter noted. 'He enjoys his work there because all the family is working and he goes there, pass the time. He doesn't do much work, but he has to be there.'

However, increasing levels of stress were evident amongst the men, particularly related to coming to terms with their decreasing levels of capacity to sustain a workload, and in some cases the unwillingness of their families to allow them to continue as they had in the past – as prime provider and head of the family. Furthermore, changing technologies are rendering the men more dependent on their children for assistance, as the following discussion in the Macedonian group illustrates:

> Lot of new things coming out. Papers you have to fill up. For everything you have to ring up. For the water. Computer things. Which is, we can't do that ... farms. Young kids farming. If you gave them a shovel and a crowbar, they worked day and night ... Now it is too much. Computers, too much writing ... Different management in orchards.
> *Q: Different from when you were younger?*
> Different management ... Computer.
> *Q: In order to order water you have to..*
> Computer.
> You are talking to the wall now.
> *Q: So these changes administration, all the modern technologies cause you a bit of heartache. Do they?*
> Oh yes.
> *Q: So how do you cope with that? What do you do?*
> Well, you ask the young ones to do the job. Because we can't do it.
> *Q: So how you feel when you have to ask a grandson to help?*
> Well, you have to ask him. No other way.
> *Q: What you said?*
> You ask him once. If he says 'No' you'll wait for the next time. When he is in good mood he will do it.
> *Q: So you have to wait for them to help you. That's what you say?*
> *So as older men, experienced men, men who have seen lot of things in your lives, haven't you, you've seen lot of changes, you've come to this country ...*
> Lot of changes.
> *Q: ... how do you feel when you can't manage on your own anymore?*
> You have to ask for help.

Long established cultural traditions of passing on values, culture, and property to following generations were experienced by the men to be under threat because of some circumstances beyond their control (economic development, changing government policy, agricultural practices, family structure and different values of the younger generations).

In relation to 'aging well', all the men saw their relationships with their families as being significant, as was being involved in some meaningful occupation or activity. For the Turkish and Macedonian men, ongoing employment or connection to the family business was especially important. For the Italians, who were perhaps more integrated with mainstream Anglo-Australian culture, seeking out alternative leisure activities (e.g. walking, bowls) was more commonly emphasized. This may be more a function of the opportunities that the men saw as being available to them.

Is it useful to think about the experiences of these men in terms of 'multiple jeopardy'? In what ways are they particularly disadvantaged according to the four elements (age, ethnicity, gender and rural location)? Are they stuck in a time warp? Are they being sidelined, suffering a loss of identity as a consequence of no longer being head of the household? Or is there another part of the picture we are missing – a more positive account of resilience and strength? Are the guiding concepts and explanatory frameworks (healthy aging, adaptation, continuity, gender, migration) limited in what they can offer us in terms of understanding the perspectives of older CALD rural men?

The importance of maintaining their role as head of the family over the life course was not of equal importance to all the men. For example, one Albanian man talked about the significant relationship with his wife and how his attitude towards his role in the family had changed over the years, particularly as his children had moved out:

> Also, because the kids have moved away from home, and you are left alone. You had children and as they move away you [him and his wife] tend to get closer. You depending more on each other opinions, decisions, all that sort of thing, all sorts of things and I think mentally that lightens the burden. And I move things that way myself. I don't want to be or to become the household or the head of the family. I don't think it work that way anymore.
>
> (Albanian male)

There was also a prevalent assumption held by many of the older men that family will be available to provide support and assistance for them as they age. However, it was evident that the support provided to the older men by other family members was not just in one direction. For example, many of the men talked about playing a caring role for their spouses.

In the Turkish group, there seemed to be an acceptance that older people will require more assistance as they age. As the Turkish interpreter noted: 'When you are young, you can deal sort of with things differently; as you get older you need more support, I think the men are getting older quickly ... They need more support from their family.' Furthermore, on account of their Muslim background, it was accepted that support would be provided by the family: 'As I get older, whoever is more active in the family helps the next person; this is also, our religion also says that, if the wife like needs help man helps the wife, if the husband needs help, wife helps.' And support is also provided by the community: 'We would like to help the family and other people around us like the family, relatives, or the friends ... To be good to them to be helpful to them' (Turkish interpreter).

Implications for health and health care

We have suggested that a life-course approach that pays cognizance to experiences of migration, gender, family and personal identity is required to properly understand the lives of older immigrant men who live in Australian rural communities. Such an approach unsettles the biomedical conception of aging, focused as it is on the biophysical body and processes of physical and mental decline. 'Healthy aging' is likely to entail much more than sustaining or restoring physical function, but rather involves physical, psychological and social well-being, including a sense of being valued and having a meaningful role with one's family and community. As with the older Turkish men described by Erol and Özbay (Chapter 9, this volume), the older Australian immigrant men whom we interviewed developed identities that are strongly linked to their 'bread-winner' role and shaped by the expectations of the 'age-appropriate masculinity' that pertain to their communities. However, as we noted, one needs to be cautious when generalizing about particular ethnic groups or ages. While gender is performed, actors tend to playfully engage with the script, with some resisting expectations of 'masculine' behaviour. Understanding the socio-cultural shaping and complexity of experiences of health and well-being is essential if health-care interventions are to be effective. In particular, there is a need to understand the diverse factors that explain why older men may neglect their health or delay seeking treatment.

Some of the service providers in this study perceived that older CALD men do not take care of their health (for example, by having regular health check-ups, taking part in health promotion activities) or seek services until they face a critical health episode.

> The only time you'll see one of these guys do something about their health is at the stage where it is an acute issue ... they have to fall over ... they have to be in significant pain before they will [go to a doctor] ... I'm talking about they've got to go to hospital in pain, they're not going to stop because it hurts they're going to stop because they've actually collapsed.
>
> (Service provider)

Some service providers attributed this reluctance to seek help to the older men's 'hard-headedness', pride and fear. They also referred to issues of communication (e.g. requiring interpreter services), lack of time and transport, the cost of health services, men's low self-awareness and associated low levels of formal education and literacy. This was perceived to affect how likely the men were able to and understand how to improve their health.

'They're not aware [older CALD men] because they've never been in the sphere, no one has ever told them about ... their health, their health is their heart, their legs, their back' (Servicer provider).

> Now can you imagine a man of perhaps my age without my schooling and perhaps my experience in life who goes to the doctor and says we have to test your prostate. What are you talking about? I don't want to be touched by you in that way. So there is a cultural barrier there which makes it very difficult. The other thing too is that a lot of the ethnic men, they tend to want to be in control.
> (Italian male community leader)

These comments convey how culture, gender, and life experiences may interact to shape individuals' understandings of health and engagements with the institutions of health care. By understanding the perspectives of the clients or potential clients of such services, this and other studies can make an important contribution towards developing a much needed and timely source of evidence-based data for policy-makers, service organizations and beyond. Service development and delivery approaches for older migrants need to be much more responsive to the significance of migration experience and identity, and the consequent community and individual needs. We have argued that engaging with older men reveals a nuanced picture of growing older, beyond one of decline and dependency, and instead adds an understanding about how the aging process changes the nature of an older man's life in various domains. Given the rapid aging of the population and the diverse communities that are and increasingly will be in need of support and care, there is an urgent need to move beyond biomedical conceptions of aging to develop perspectives that are more attentive to the contexts of people's lives. While we do not deny that biophysical changes accompany aging, we contend that there is a need for policy-makers and practitioners to recognize that definitions and experiences of aging are profoundly shaped by culture and, as such, are subject to change. Health-care policies and strategies that focus on improving services while neglecting the factors that lie beyond biomedicine and the institutions of health care that affect outlooks and behaviour, we suggest, are likely to be of limited value.

References

Addis, M., and Mahalik, J. (2003) 'Men, masculinity, and the contexts of help seeking', *American Psychologist,* 58: 5–14.
Angus, J., and Reeve, P. (2006) 'Ageism: A threat to "aging well" in the 21st century', *Journal of Applied Gerontology,* 25: 137–52.
Arber, S., and Ginn, J. (1995) *Connecting Gender and Ageing: A Sociological Approach,* Buckingham: Open University Press.
Arber, S., Davidson, K., and Ginn, J. (eds) (2003) *Gender and Ageing: Changing Roles and Relationships,* Maidenhead: Open University Press.

Archer, L. (2003) *Race, Masculinity and Schooling: Muslim Boys and Education*, Maidenhead: Open University Press.
Atchley, R. (1989) 'A continuity theory of normal aging', *The Gerontologist*, 29: 183–90.
Atchley, R. (1998) 'Activity adaptations to the development of functional limitations and results for subjective well-being in later adulthood: A qualitative analysis of longitudinal panel data over a 16-year period', *Journal of Aging Studies*, 12: 19–38.
Atchley, R. C. (1999) *Continuity and Adaptation in Aging: Creating Positive Experiences*, Baltimore, MD: Johns Hopkins University Press.
Australian Bureau of Statistics (2011) *Migration, Australia, 2009–10. Cat no. 3412.0*, Canberra: Commonwealth of Australia.
Australian Institute of Health and Welfare (2010) *A Snapshot of Men's Health in Regional and Remote Australia*, Canberra: Australian Government
Baltes, M. M. (1996) *The Many Faces of Dependency in Old Age*, Cambridge: Cambridge University Press.
Baltes, P. B., and Smith, J. (1999) 'Multilevel and systemic analyses of old age: Theoretical and empirical evidence for a fourth age', in V. L. Bengtson and K.W. Schaie (eds), *Handbook of Theories of Aging* (pp. 153–173), New York: Springer.
Bambling, M., Kavanagh, D., Lewis, G., King, R., King, D., Sturk, H., Turpin, M., Gallois, C., and Bartlett, H. (2007) 'Challenges faced by general practitioners and allied mental health services in providing mental health services in rural Queensland', *Australian Journal of Rural Health*, 15: 126–30.
Bengston, V. L., Elder, G. H., and Putney, N. M. (2005) 'The lifecourse perspective on ageing: Linked lives, timing and history', in M. L. Johnson (ed.), *The Cambridge Handbook of Age and Ageing* (pp. 493–501), Cambridge: Cambridge University Press.
Calasanti, T., and Slevin, K. F. (eds) (2006) *Age Matters: Re-aligning Feminist Thinking*, New York: Routledge.
Constant, A., Gataullina, L., and Zimmermann, K. F. (2006) 'Gender, ethnic identity and work', *Discussion Paper 2420*, November, IZA: Bonn.
Council on the Ageing (2008) *A Strategic Policy Framework for Older Men's Health* Melbourne, Victoria: Council on the Ageing.
Courtenay, W. H. (2000) 'Constructions of masculinity and their influence on men's wellbeing: A theory of gender and health', *Social Science and Medicine*, 50: 1385–1401.
Crowther, M. R., Parker, M. W., Achenbaum, W. A., Larimore, W. L., and Koenig, H. G. (2002) 'Rowe and Kahn's model of successful aging revisited: Positive spirituality. The forgotten factor', *The Gerontologist*, 42: 613–20.
Department of Health and Ageing (2008) *Developing a Men's Health Policy for Australia*, Canberra: Australian Government.
Faircloth, C. A. (ed.) (2003) *Aging Bodies: Images and Everyday Experience*, Walnut Creek, CA: AltaMira Press.
Feldman, S., and Seedsman, T. (2005) 'Family: Changing families, changing times', in M. Poole (ed.), *Ageing: New Choices, New Challenges*. Crows Nest, NSW: Allen & Unwin.
Fishman, J. R. (2010) 'The making of viagra: The biomedicalization of sexual dysfunction', in A. E. Clarke, L. Mamo, J. R. Fosket, J. R. Fishman, and J. K. Shim (eds), *Biomedicalization: Technoscience, Health and Illness* (pp. 289–306), Durham, NC, and London: Duke University Press.

Fuller, J., Edwards, J., Proeter, N., and Moss, J. (2000) 'How definition of mental health problems can influence help seeking in rural and remote communities', *Australian Journal of Rural Health,* 8: 148–53.
Galdas, P. M. (2009) 'Men, masculinity and help-seeking', in A. Broom and T. Tovey (eds), *Men's Health: Body, Identity and Social Context* (63–82), Southern Gate, Chichester: Wiley-Blackwell.
Gilleard, C., and Higgs, P. (2005) *Contexts of Ageing: Class, Cohort and Community,* Cambridge: Polity Press.
Granville, G., and Evandrou, M. (2010) 'Older men, work and health', *Occupational Medicine,* 60: 178–83.
Jensen, H., Munk, K., and Madsen, S. (2010) 'Gendering late-life depression? The coping process in a group of elderly men', *Nordic Psychology,* 62: 56–80.
Kiropoulos, L. A., Blashki, G., and Klimidis, S. (2005) 'Managing mental illness in patients from CALD backgrounds', *Australian Family Physician,* 34: 259–64.
Kraaij, V., Arensman, E., and Spinhoven, P. (2002) 'Negative life events and depression in elderly persons: A meta-analysis', *Journals of Gerontology Series B: Psychological Sciences and Social Sciences,* 57: 87–94.
Larkin, M. (2001) 'Robert Butler: Championing a healthy view of ageing', *The Lancet,* 357: 48.
Loe, M. (2004) *The Rise of Viagra: How the Little Blue Pill Changed Sex in America,* New York and London: New York University Press.
McCann Mortimer, P., Ward, L., and Winefield, H. (2008) 'Successful ageing by whose definition? Views of older, spiritually affiliated women', *Australasian Journal of Ageing,* 27: 200–4.
McDonald, L. (2011) 'Theorising about ageing, family and immigration', *Ageing and Society,* 31: 1180–1201.
Maynard, M., Afshar, H., Franks, M., and Wray, S. (2008) *Women in Later Life : Exploring Race and Ethnicity,* Maidenhead: Open University Press.
Petersen, A. (1998) *Unmasking the Masculine: 'Men' and 'Identity' in a Sceptical Age,* London: Sage.
Pugh, R., Scharf, T., Williams, C., and Roberts, R. (2007) *Obstacles to Using and Providing Rural Social Care* (Research Briefing, 22), London: Social Care Institute for Excellence.
Radermacher, H., Feldman, S., and Browning, C. (2009) 'Mainstream versus ethno-specific community aged care services: It's not an "either or"', *Australasian Journal on Ageing,* 28: 58–63.
Reiger, K. (2005) 'History: The rise of the modern institution', in M. Poole (ed.), *Family: Changing Families, Changing Times* (pp. 43–65), Crows Nest, NSW: Allen & Unwin.
Rowe, J., and Kahn, R. L. (1998) *Successful Ageing,* New York: Dell Publishing.
Rowland, D. (1991) *Ageing in Australia: Population Trends and Social Issues,* Sydney: Longman Cheshire.
Saracci, R. (1997) 'The World Health Organization needs to reconsider its definition of health', *British Medical Journal,* 314: 1409–10.
Sweeney, P., and Kisely, S. (2003) 'Barriers to managing mental health in Western Australia', *Australian Journal of Rural Health,* 11: 205–10.
Thompson, E. (1994) 'Older men as invisible in contemporary society', in E. Thompson (ed.), *Older Men's Lives* (pp. 1–21), Thousand Oaks, CA: Sage.

Tohit, N., Browning, C., and Radermacher, H. (2012) 'We want a peaceful life here and hereafter: Healthy ageing perspectives of older Malays in Malaysia', *Ageing & Society*, 32: 404–424.

Torres, S. (2004) 'Making sense of the construct of successful ageing: the migrant experience', in S. O. Daatland and S. Biggs (eds), *Ageing and Diversity: Multiple Pathways and Cultural Migrations* (pp. 125–140), Bristol: Policy Press.

Vaillant, G. E. (2002) *Ageing Well: Surprising Guideposts to a Happier Life from the Landmark Harvard Study of Adult Development*, Carlton North, Victoria: Scribe Publications.

Vaillant, G. E., and Mukamal, K. (2001) 'Successful aging', *American Journal of Psychiatry*, 158: 839–47.

Vincent, J. A. (2003) *Old Age*, London and New York: Routledge.

Vincent, J. A. (2008) 'The cultural construction of old age as a biological phenomenon: Science and anti-ageing technologies', *Journal of Aging Studies*, 22: 331–9.

West, C., and Zimmerman, D. H. (1987) 'Doing gender', *Gender and Society*, 1: 125–51.

World Health Organization (1952) *Constitution of the World Health Organization*, Geneva: World Health Organization.

World Health Organization (2011) *Redefining 'Health'*: www.who.int/bulletin/bulletin_board/83/ustun11051/en (accessed Nov. 2011).

6 What a difference a gay makes

The constitution of the 'older gay man'

William Leonard, Duane Duncan and Catherine Barrett

Old age ain't no place for sissies.

(Bette Davis)

Introduction

There's an *old* joke in gay circles that 30 years in gay time is the equivalent of 80 years in straight time: gay men, it seems, are over the hill by the time they hit 30! The joke conjures, as it parodies, a common stereotype of gay men and commercial gay culture, ageist and youth-obsessed, even as it highlights the ways in which being gay is constituted in relation to a heterosexual norm. However this joke is read, it captures the exceptionalism of being gay that is still part of many gay men's lives: sexual oddities within an overwhelmingly heterosexual, if not heterosexist, culture. This exceptionalism may be waning for a new generation of gay and queer young men, at a time when support for same-sex marriage and equal love is on the rise and gay issues are being mainstreamed in many Western countries (Gardiner 2011; Victorian Government Department of Health 2009).[1] But for many middle-aged and older gay men, feelings of exceptionalism have framed their sense of who and what they are, and their place, or lack thereof, in the culture at large.

Much of the research and policy on men's health and well-being has assumed a heterosexual, male subject for whom gender is the major determinant of aging. The emerging men's health agenda has relied, heavily, on feminist theorizations of gender as a relation of social inequality. While the women's health movement has used this critical understanding of gender to challenge women's social subordination and champion their specific health needs, it is only recently that a men's health movement has begun to explore the ways in which gender also operates to compromise men's health and well-being (Gregory *et al.* 2006).[2]

A narrow focus on gender in men's health marginalizes gay men and their particular experiences of aging. Furthermore, it ignores the ways in which gender is itself implicated in sexuality and how the two interact to produce more complicated and variegated patterns of health and aging *among* men. As queer theorists have convincingly argued, in Western, liberal democracies heterosexism operates as a regulatory system aimed at securing a singular, hetero-normative relationship between sex, gender and sexuality (Butler 1991; Sedgwick 1990). Heterosexism assumes that men, that is 'real' men, are born male, exhibit masculine behaviours, and are attracted, exclusively, to those of the opposite sex. Men who depart from these norms, including effeminate and gay men, are subject to varying levels of discrimination and abuse (Leonard 2005; Sedgwick 1994).

This chapter deploys this more complex, *queer* understanding of the co-implication of sex, gender and sexuality in its exploration of gay men's experiences of aging. It focuses on the ways in which biomedical technologies that target the aging gay male body necessarily draw on, even as they question, heterosexist constructions of sexuality and gender, and the relationship between the two.

The chapter is built around a number of discrete but overlapping concerns. How have gay men's experiences of aging and gay male embodiment been influenced by changing attitudes towards homosexuality and gender? What has been the impact of the medicalization of male aging on gay men's lives? How do biotechnologies that take sexual attractiveness and potency as markers of successful male aging refashion dominant stereotypes of both gay and heterosexual men and complicate the gendered divisions between the two? And finally, how does the biotechnological and social reorganization of aged care services impact on the health and well-being of an older cohort of gay men?

Where are the older gay men? Competing fictions and a farewell to stereotypes

There is very little empirical research that investigates the relationships between biomedicine, aging and gay men to draw on. Rather, research on gay men and aging has tended to emphasize the generational and cohort effects of gay identity on men's aging, including a focus on the social exclusions experienced by older gay men, and a concern with heterosexism in policy and services for older gay, lesbian and bisexual people (Rosenfeld 2010).[3] According to Bauer *et al.* (2007) materials on sexuality and aging are generally produced for nursing and healthcare workers and focus, primarily, on surveys exploring older people's sexual behaviour and knowledge, healthcare providers' attitudes towards older people *as* sexual beings, and the impact of illness on sexual behaviour and relationships. Scherrer (2009: 7) notes that the gerontological literature has begun to present sexual activity in older age as a natural, even fundamental, component of 'healthy aging'. Researchers who are critical of widely held beliefs that growing older is a process of sexual decline, culminating in old age as a period of celibacy if not asexuality, nonetheless often share with those they criticize an unstated assumption that the sexual life and practices in question are heterosexual. As Rosenfeld (2010) argues, while heterosexuality is rarely named as such in gerontological literature, it is nonetheless assumed in discussions of family, sexual activity, care-giving and social support.

The failure of these materials to engage with the range of issues facing gay men (and other sexual minorities) reflects a heterosexual bias or conceit within the research on aging more broadly. Accompanying the shift in awareness about the importance of sexuality to health and well-being are a range of biotechnologies and expert discourses that suggest successful aging starts in mid-life and rests on individuals adopting 'healthy' practices aimed at optimizing their sexual performance and well-being into older age (Cardrona 2008; Katz and Marshall 2003). The cultural imagery and invitation to remain sexually active that accompany these discourses have been critiqued for reinforcing conservative notions of heterosexuality and gender (Katz and Marshall 2003; Potts *et al.* 2006). Performance enhancing drugs, of which Viagra is perhaps the best known, are marketed to men as a means of ensuring their continued sexual potency and attractiveness to women. Cosmetic surgeries and body-image enhancing techniques, once the exclusive prerogative of women, are now marketed to both sexes, as a means of ensuring their continued *reciprocal* attraction well into older age.

However, consideration of gay men within mainstream research on aging has rarely moved beyond a fascination with very narrow and deeply problematic stereotypes of homosexuality (Fredriksen-Goldsen and Muraco 2010; Haber 2009; Lo 2006). These stereotypes have their origins in medical and popular discourses of the late nineteenth and early twentieth centuries, which depicted homosexuality, variously, as a sin, illness or sexual perversion (Altman 1971; Dollimore 1991).

The term 'homosexuality' was first used in the medical and research literature by the sexologist Richard von Kraft-Ebbing in 1886 (Weeks 1985). The early sexologists sought to develop a scientific taxonomy of human sexuality and, more pointedly, of the sexual perversions. Homosexuality was classified as a form of sexual inversion with male homosexuals understood to exhibit feminine behaviours, which, in turn, underpinned both their choice of sexual object and sexual acts (Ellis and Abarbanel 1961: 485). Male homosexuality became a code word for sexual perversion writ large. 'Homosexuality may be associated with other perversions', warned the authors of *The Encycolpaedia of Sexual Behaviour*, 'such as exhibitionism, sadism, neurosis, insanity or alcoholism'. 'Homosexuality', they concluded, 'is socially important because it may involve or lead to other offenses … assaults on young boys by school masters … and prostitution … in large cities' (Ellis and Abarbanel 1961: 808).

According to the plot lines of this popular medical fiction, heterosexual men are destined to grow old swaddled in a web of social and familial relationships. However, no such fate awaited the male homosexual. Defined and governed solely by his sexual desire, and adrift in a sea of fleeting and uncommitted sexual relationships, the aging homosexual was bound for a sad and lonely end. 'The homosexual rarely builds up a home or permanent circle of friends', wrote Allen, a consulting psychiatrist in 1961 (quoted in Hughes 2006: 54), '[w]hatever the causes, the homosexual often ends up lonely'. More worrying was the implication that older gay men, 'having lost [their] physical attractiveness and sexual appeal to the young men [they] crave', become sexual predators who prey on the vulnerable and the very young (Kelly 1977: 329).

From the outset, however, homosexual men challenged the veracity of these discourses. By the 1920s there were thriving queer subcultures in Paris and Berlin and by the late 1940s and early 1950s gay and lesbian bars and clubs were appearing in urban centres across the US (Faderman 1991; Halperin 1990). These subcultures provided the necessary communal spaces and human capital for the birth of gay liberation in the 1960s and 1970s.

As numerous queer commentators have argued, gay liberation constituted a counter or reverse discourse, appropriating and *inverting* both the meaning and value of dominant medical and popular constructions of homosexuality (Foucault 1988; Didier 2001). This is perhaps best captured in the title of Dennis Altman's 1971 gay manifesto, *Homosexual: Oppression and Liberation*. Gay liberation appropriated the very terms of the oppressor, giving them a new and positive twist. In so doing, it rejected the hegemony of medical and scientific authority and with it dominant and empty stereotypes of gay men as degenerate, perverse or ill.

Gay liberation, in turn, assisted in the birth of an open and publicly visible commercial gay culture, one defined as much by an ethos of sexual pleasure as by collective pride. Commercial gay culture brought with it new and different types of gay masculinity. By the early 1980s, the beefy-but-muscular, moustachioed clone had become the poster boy of gay male identity (Cole 2000). On the one hand, the clone represented a direct challenge to medical and popular depictions of gay men as inverts, effeminate and camp. On the other, it bought into conservative constructions of gender, with gay men out*manning* heterosexual men in the performance of their masculinity. Following Connell, the clone became the hegemonic or dominant expression of masculinity within a competing sea of gay masculinities that included twinks, muscle Marys, camp and drag (Connell 2005; Connell and Messerschmidt 2005).

Despite a further three decades of gay and queer activism, which has seen not only the advent of HIV and AIDS but also the continued growth and diversification of commercial gay culture and new ways of 'being and doing gay' (Dowsett 1996), the limited mainstream research on gay men and aging has yet to move beyond the gravitational pull of the 'aging homosexual' stereotypes. Fredriksen-Goldsen and Muraco (2010: 397), in their review of twenty-five years of research on sexuality and aging, conclude 'Contrary to the stereotype, the majority of early articles describe positive psychological functioning among older gay men and lesbians.' 'Older gay men and lesbian adults', they continue, 'are not isolated but have various means of support' (2010: 400). These conclusions are supported by similar reviews by Haber (2009) and Lo (2006).

These reviews detail alternate, 'positive' models of gay aging in the research literature, in which older gay men's experiences of exclusion and discrimination are sources of resilience and strength. Haber (2009: 256), for example, argues that 'the current cohort of elder gay men' is subject to 'a unique double jeopardy ... being gay in a world of heterosexual supremacy ... [and] being older in a GLBT [gay, lesbian bisexual and transgender] community that values youth'. Older gay men are doubly marginalized, ostracized from the mainstream by virtue of their homosexuality and from commercial gay culture by virtue of their age. According to the terms of this analysis, successful gay male aging is a process of 'crisis management', learning, as Fredriksen-Goldsen and Muraco (2010: 397) put it, to transfer the skills gained in the 'management of one stigmatised identity early in the life course (e.g. gay, lesbian, bisexual) ... to the successful management of a later stigmatized identity'.

That all these reviews rely on an assessment of the degree to which nearly three decades of research on gay men and aging supports or contradicts narrow, if not archaic, medical stereotypes is testimony to the ongoing influence of these stereotypes and medical authority on research and popular perceptions of gay men and aging. Furthermore, the alternate models of gay male aging that they profile replay many of the deeper, problematic assumptions of the professional discourses these models are intended to critique. Whether or not the totality of gay men's lives is reduced to an expression of an aberrant sexuality or a symptom of heterosexist discrimination and abuse, the research literature on gay men's aging has yet to escape the shadow cast by dominant medical and popular stereotypes of homosexuality and the 'old queen' (Kelly 1977: 329).

This singular focus on stereotypes forecloses a raft of research questions that do not fit within its narrow orbit. It precludes detailed analyses of the ways in which the increasing legal and social recognition of sexual and gender identity minorities in Western democracies impacts on an older cohort of gay men's experiences of aging. It also precludes consideration of how this period of rapid and intense social change has led to very different experiences of aging among different age cohorts of gay men (Jones and Pugh 2005; Heaphy 2007; Robinson 2008).

Furthermore, as others have noted (Cronin and King 2010; Heaphy 2007; Heaphy *et al.* 2004), there is also a danger in conceiving of gay men as a homogeneous group who share a unitary, non-heterosexual experience of aging. This overlooks the ways in which gender, ethnicity, opportunity and wealth play out differently for different groups of gay men and their experiences of aging in relation to the techno-scientific claims of biomedicine. Finally, a failure to look at how the heterosexual/homosexual binary underpins the naturalizing claims of biomedicine with regard to masculinity and aging reinforces the authority of those discourses, while overlooking the parallels between heterosexual and gay men's experiences of aging.

Consuming sex – biomedicine, gay men and body image

The advent of HIV and AIDS in the 1980s radically altered the public expression and embodiment of gay male identity. Images of the ravaged and prematurely aged AIDS body had the contradictory effects of consolidating a nascent gay community against the spread of the HIV virus while, at the same time, reconstituting the gay male body as a site of social anxiety and bio-regulation. In the popular imagination, gay men were transformed from sexual deviants and predators into the harbingers of disease and death. As Patton (1996: 117) put it, the AIDS epidemic led to reactive public health policies aimed at ensuring that HIV 'didn't leak from its subcultural [gay] spaces into the mainstream'.

In countries like Australia, researchers and policy-makers, in partnership with gay community organizations, developed a *calculus of sexual risk* both to minimize HIV infection among gay men and limit the spread of the virus into the 'population at large' (Leonard and Mitchell 2000; Sendziuk 2003). While gay community agencies increasingly focused on developing a safe-sex culture among gay men, this emerging biomedical discourse reconstituted men-who-have-sex-with-men as little more than vectors for the possible transmission of the HIV virus (Dowsett 1996; Leonard in press).

With the advent of highly active antiretroviral therapies (HAART) in the mid-1990s gay men's lives underwent yet another radical change. In those jurisdictions where medications are accessible, and in some cases state-subsidized, HAART has given HIV-positive gay men the opportunity to live longer and healthier lives. For a younger cohort of gay and queer young men, HAART has meant that they no longer view HIV infection as a death sentence, but, rather, as a manageable, long-term, chronic condition (Elford 2006; Halkitis, Zade, *et al.* 2004).

If HIV and AIDS opened gay men's sexual lives to new forms of state-regulated biomedical surveillance, HAART can, perhaps, be understood as one of the first, medically authorized, anti-aging technologies to target the male body. HAART intervened to halt the premature aging that accompanied AIDS. It not only extended the lives of HIV-positive gay men but also shifted public interest away from a morbid fascination with the AIDS body *in extremis*. In so doing, HAART helped unpick a decade's association between gay men, HIV/AIDS and death.

The increasing biomedicalization of gay male sexual practices and of HIV-positive, gay male aging that followed in the wake of HIV and AIDS was accompanied by radical shifts within gay community, culture and identity. By the late 1980s and early 1990s, the increasing legal and social recognition of sexual and gender identity minorities fuelled the growth and diversification of commercial gay culture. As gay men became more publicly confident and 'out', they developed their own neighbourhoods, pubs, clubs, associations and events. The commercial gay scene provided a wide range of clearly and publicly identified sites and venues where gay men could socialize and 'sexualize' *as* gay men (Leonard in press), bringing with it an increased emphasis on body image and appearance.

One of the key elements of commercial gay culture has been the commodification of the male body and with it those body-image-enhancing practices that increase physical and sexual attractiveness and promise to minimize, if not overcome, aging and its effects (Bordo 1999; Cole 2000). The rise of a commercial gay culture has underwritten notions of the 'pink economy' where gay men are positioned as idealized consumers and trendsetters (Bell and Binnie 2000; Jones and Pugh 2005). This not only ignores socio-economic diversity within the gay male community. It also underscores the degree to which gay male identities are no longer dependent on medical and psychological discourses alone, but also on the processes of late consumer capitalism for their articulation and visibility.

Further, commercial gay culture has provided a fertile ground for the expansion of cosmetic goods and services once targeted exclusively at women (Bordo 1999). The gay liberationist ethos which celebrated sexuality and pleasure has proven to be a productive basis on which to sell gay men products and technologies designed to bring them closer to the promises of sexual freedom. These include designer clothes, body-grooming techniques and weight-loss procedures, and biomedical technologies, such as hormone replacement, collagen and botox injections, and plastic surgery.

In part, gay men's uptake of these products and technologies reflects the historical association, in medical and popular discourse, between femininity and homosexuality (Butler 1991; Garber 1992). More complex, however, are the ways in which gay men have appropriated hegemonic forms of masculinity as a challenge to the medical and popular discourses of inversion that circulated prior to gay liberation. In the process, commercial gay culture has facilitated the commercialization of masculinity in all its forms, providing a market for cosmetic goods and services targeting heterosexual men of varying ages (Bordo 1999; Simpson 1994). However, as heterosexual men take up the body grooming techniques and anti-aging biotechnologies first adopted by gay men, they too, are subject to the pressure to maintain their sexual attractiveness and potency as a demonstration of 'healthy' aging (Katz 2010; Katz and Marshall 2003).

In-between men and healthy aging

It could be argued that new aging is indebted to the biomedicalization and commodification of the gay male body. The AIDS epidemic reconstituted a class of men, gay men, as an object of biomedical regulation and surveillance. At the same time, this class of men became a conduit through which a range of body-image enhancing technologies, traditionally associated with women, could be marketed to men *en masse*, irrespective, or in spite of, their sexual orientation. For gay men, these technologies were those that focused on sexual pleasure and performance, and held the promise of maintaining the sexual attractiveness and capacity of the male body as it aged.

New aging has expanded the biomedical gaze beyond a class of men defined by their sexuality and relationship to a particular illness. It has rebadged the continuation of sexual activity into older age, not as a sign of sexual excess, but rather as a marker of healthy aging (Katz 2010; Katz and Marshall 2003). In so doing, it has taken those biotechnologies and cosmetic procedures that commercial gay culture promotes as part of gay men's sexual repertoire and self-presentation and drawn them under the banner and protection of 'healthy' male aging.

The repackaging of sex and sexual activity as key indicators of healthy aging has had an impact both on gay men's understandings and experiences of aging, and on the complex relationships between gay and heterosexual men and the commercialization of biomedical anti-aging technologies. Among gay men, it has highlighted both the youth-centred focus of commercial gay culture and how recent history impacts differently on different age cohorts of gay men and their relationship to anti-aging technologies (Robinson 2008; Jones and Pugh 2005). At the same time, new aging has questioned, even as it reasserts, many of the stereotypes on which the heterosexist division between gay and straight men depends.

Robinson (2008), in his ethnographic study of gay male aging in Australia, argues that different age cohorts of gay men have very different, if not incommensurate, understandings of what it means to be male and gay. As Jones and Pugh (2005: 249) put it, 'being young and gay today is very different from the experiences of older gay men'. Middle-aged gay men are likely to have a very different relationship to their bodies as they age, compared with gay men now aged in their 70s and 80s. While the older cohort have lived through recent advances in anti-aging biotechnologies, their embodiment as male and gay is likely to have been shaped by the deeply homophobic popular and professional discourses of the early to mid twentieth century (Jones and Pugh 2005; Robinson 2008). In contrast, the middle-aged and younger cohorts have 'come out' at a time when discrimination is on the wane and commercial gay culture is providing new forms of male embodiment no longer defined in opposition to mainstream constructions of masculinity and aging.

For many gay men, aging within the confines of commercial gay culture is experienced as a double-edged sword. On the one hand, gay men describe ageism within the 'scene' which requires serious financial and time commitments to anti-aging and body-image-enhancing technologies. On the other, they describe the benefits of greater attention to appearance and exercise and with that, the deferment of the physical decline perceived to impact heterosexual men at an earlier age (Slevin and Linneman 2010; Robinson 2008). As one of the middle-aged respondents in Duncan's (2009) study of gay men's embodied identities commented:

> We've understood health and a healthy lifestyle more than [heterosexual men] probably have. You know, you don't have to let yourself go. There's some very stylish, very sexy older gay men.

Another participant expressed a similarly optimistic (and competitive) view of growing older:

> I'm not so concerned about aging and losing what I have. In that respect I'm actually proud of the fact that I actually have this understanding so that when I age I'm hopefully going to look better than someone who has aged as well but hasn't had the experience or knowledge that I've had in terms of looking after myself.

For these gay men, 'successful aging' was measured more by the maintenance of the body's appearance than by its function, performance or even its durability in the face of wear and tear. These men derived a sense of power and control from the assumption that they would age better than other gay and heterosexual men of a similar age. Furthermore, these gay men perceived their choices to be freely available, and thus freely made, without reflecting on the way those choices may embody powerful cultural norms and require the ongoing disciplining of their bodies into old age, and beyond (Bordo 1999; Petersen 2007). The solutions offered by exercise, diet and lifestyle expressed by these men indicate the ways in which physical decline has come to be understood as aging itself (Vincent 2009; Cardrona 2008; Powell *et al.* 2006). Indeed, these respondents expressed confidence in the ability of technical, medical and pharmaceutical products to provide individualized solutions not only to the biological processes of aging but also to the hierarchical and ageist organization of the commercial gay scene.

One of the potentially positive implications of new aging discourses where sexuality is understood to be an aspect of every person's health and well-being is that the invisibility of older gay men is perhaps less sustainable. However, the association between healthy aging and continued sexual activity, combined with commercial gay culture's emphasis on youth and body image, put increased pressures on gay men to avail themselves of the full range of anti-aging technologies, from cosmetics to demanding physical regimes and invasive surgeries. According to Robinson (2008: 176), the primary purpose of the commercial gay scene 'is as a sexual market for young or *youthful* men' (emphasis added) 'and its attractions' he concludes, 'appeal less to men as they grow older'. Clearly, for those gay men whose sense of identity and social life is wedded to the commercial scene, the pressure to maintain a *youthful* appearance increases with age, as does their dependence on, and belief in the efficacy of, anti-aging biotechnologies. Gay men who refuse or are unable to engage in those well-being and self-care practices espoused by the market are likely to find themselves excluded from the commercial gay scene, *and* from progressive understandings of gay sexuality that reside in conservative definitions of masculinity.

At the same time, however, new aging threatens to reassert some of the most problematic stereotypes of gay men on which the heterosexist divisions between gay and straight depend. If, as Katz and Marshall (2003: 11) persuasively argue, 'the discourses of positive aging have created the sexy, ageless consumer as a personally and socially responsible citizen' that citizen is imagined, in the main, as heterosexual. The rebadging of technologies associated with gay men's sexual pleasure under the banner of healthy male aging divests those technologies of any association with the commonly perceived excesses of gay sexuality. Dildos can be rebadged as 'prostate stimulation devices' for a mainstream audience suffering the deflating effects of prostate surgery. Viagra is marketed to men as a way of managing the debilitating effects of erectile dysfunction and ensuring the maintenance of healthy, heterosexual relationships and not as an adjunct to stimulants that enable men to maintain their erections during periods of prolonged sexual engagement with one or more partners.

Under the imprimatur of health, new aging leaves out the myriad of sexual practices, performances and identities that cannot be wrapped 'in the aura of respectability' that it uses to market itself (Katz and Marshall 2003: 11). If new aging offers a range of biotechnologies to counter the effects of aging on sexual performance, the sexuality that is being buttressed is constituted as both heterosexual *and* natural. This is consistent with Gayle Rubin's notion of the sex hierarchy (1984) in which those sexual practices whose primary aim is pleasure, and which exist beyond the orbit of family, monogamy and reproduction, are considered unnatural or abnormal. Yet Rubin's hierarchy is not a static principle. The acceptability of new pleasures, and the marginalization of others, is part of a political process through which gender relations may be reordered, and new gendered hierarchies established. Biomedicine in regard to aging and masculinity shifts the line between natural and unnatural sexuality under the guise of health. In so doing, it creates new alliances between gay and heterosexual men.

For example, reproductive biotechnologies are reworking the sexualized *and* gendered divisions between the natural and the unnatural. For those gay male couples who have both the desire and capital to access IVF and surrogacy, there is the opportunity to enter the orbit of family and reproduction, and with that, access to familial structures of aging previously reserved for heterosexual men. This entry, however, threatens to introduce a new division between responsible and irresponsible gay men, between those who are willing to subordinate their sexual excesses to a familial narrative of reproduction and monogamy, and those who are not. This division threatens to move beyond the orbit of excessive gay male sexuality to include new forms of marginalized masculinities more broadly, men, who in various ways and for various reasons, continue to *invert* the dominant sexual hierarchy by putting sexual pleasure above reproductive desire.

Older gay men and care settings

The reassertion of negative stereotypes of gay men is perhaps nowhere more evident and forceful than in the provision and delivery of aged and community care services. For an older cohort of gay men, the prospect of various forms of dependency on aged care raises the spectre of *a return to the closet* where their quality of care and capacity to be open about their sexuality depend on the beliefs and values of service providers towards homosexuality.

A recent Australian state-based survey, exploring aged-care services providers' knowledge of HIV, found that many would assume that a client who identified as gay would also be HIV-positive (Cummins *et al.* 2010). This was highlighted in another Australian study by Barrett (2008) who found that aged care service providers had little knowledge of HIV/AIDS or how to provide appropriate care to gay male clients. As one carer of a particular gay client said:

> We don't have any information on whether he has AIDS. I feel sorry for the poor personal care attendants that go in there and don't wear gloves to protect themselves. If they get AIDS who are they going to sue?

Research in Australia and the UK also suggests that most aged-care service providers do not believe they have any gay, lesbian, bisexual or transgender clients and that very few understand the pressure such clients are under *not* to reveal their sexual orientation (GRAI and Curtin 2010). Furthermore, as Barrett *et al.* (2009) show, the assumption that aging is a process of sexual decline can doubly disadvantage older gay men who, in the process of being 'desexed', are also 'degayed'. One such example is provided in a focus group with nursing home staff who described the admission of a new resident who 'used to be gay' (ibid. 36). A further example is provided by 'Tom', a 64-year-old HIV-positive gay man in a nursing home who said:

> I can't be a gay man [here]. I miss the intimacy of male company. I'm in a nursing home, it's not my real home, there's no privacy here. I'm not able to live a gay man's life in a nursing home.
>
> (Barrett 2008: 57)[4]

A recent UK report (Guasp 2011) found that almost half of GLBT respondents would be uncomfortable revealing their sexual identity to home care staff and would not access services they need because of anticipated discrimination. This figure jumps to nearly 90 per cent in a US study of GLBT respondents (and their supporters) in aged care facilities who reported that did not feel safe enough to disclose their sexual orientation or gender identity (National Senior Citizens Law Center *et al.* 2011).

The consequences of the resurfacing of stereotypes of gay men in the context of aged and community care is that many older gay men delay or avoid such services for fear that disclosure will result in discrimination and reduced quality of services. For those older gay men already receiving services, the pressure from prejudiced staff to deny who they are and how they love is at odds with the new aging and its promotion of active sexual expression as a component of healthy aging. It is also an affront to their dignity and humanity. To adapt Bette Davis, aged care ain't no place for sissies.

Conclusion

Perhaps more so than any other group of Western men in the last century, gay men have experienced enormous social change in regard to medicine, masculinity and aging. Prior to the 1960s, it was possible to be imprisoned or hospitalized for being homosexual or engaging in same-sex activity. For men of these generations, the experience of identifying as a gay man was one shaped by medical, religious and psychological understandings of homosexuality that predate gay liberation. In contrast, for a younger generation of gay men, the possibility of same-sex marriage and parenthood seem tantalizingly inevitable, even as conventions around family life and intimacy in many Western democracies continue to splinter.

Much of the established research on gay men and aging has tended to explore the implications of these changes for different cohorts of men, particularly in regard to the effects and accuracy of stereotypes which originated in medical and psychological discourses from the early–mid twentieth century. The relationship between gay and heterosexual men's experiences of aging have generally not been addressed. Yet discussion of new aging reveals the limitations of conceiving of gay and straight men's experiences of aging as separate and independent processes. At one level, commercial gay culture has acted as a conduit between the sex-segregated worlds of heterosexual men and women, with heterosexual men increasingly invited to adopt many of the body-image-enhancing technologies previously associated with, if not definitive of, femininity. 'New aging for the straight guy' has relied, in large part, on marketing many of the technologies (and anxieties) associated with gay men to a mainstream male audience, under the banner of 'healthy' aging.

This has involved an expansion of what might be considered acceptable masculine practices and, as Marshall and Katz (2003) have argued, relies heavily on the naturalization of sexuality as a function of health and personal responsibility. Yet, paradoxically, the renaturalizing claims of these technologies and practices, insofar as they seek to 'remedy' the failings of the 'natural' male body, mean that the sexual opportunities being opened up may further entrench definitions of masculinity as founded on characteristics of virility, strength and penetrative heterosexual practice. In so doing, they reproduce conservative definitions of masculinity, particularly in relation to heterosexual gender relations. Privileging heterosexual practice as the natural basis upon which healthy masculinity is defined, reinstates homosexuality as the constitutive outside to heterosexuality.

However, gay men are unlikely to see themselves excluded from the invitation to engage in the anti-aging strategies being increasingly promoted to heterosexual men, given that these messages are consistent with the imperatives of the commercial gay scene. Those gay men with the right financial and corporeal capital may, in fact, increase their broader social capital by adhering to the stylized images of aging being promoted in anti-aging materials for men. Yet, the implicit costs of this bargain remain the stigmatization of 'lesser' men, including those who fail to take responsibility for their aging, those who 'let themselves go' and those whose sexual practices subvert the 'aura of respectability' in which these new pleasures of the flesh are clothed.

Notes

1 According to Galaxy polling the percentage of Australians who supported marriage equality jumped from 38 percent in 2004 to 62 percent in 2010. In 2010, 80 percent of young Australians aged 18 to 24 years supported marriage equality. At www.australianmarriageequality.com/wp (accessed Aug. 2011). The Victorian Government, for example, has produced a set of guidelines for the delivery of gay, lesbian, bisexual, transgender and intersex (GLBTI) sensitive mainstream health and human services. See Victorian Government Department of Health (2009).
2 In particular, the men's health movement has been concerned with the ways in which hegemonic or dominant constructions of masculinity have worked to reduce men's health-seeking behaviours and put them at increased risk of a range of health problems compared to women. See the *Medical Journal of Australia's* special issue on men's health and the introduction, Gregory *et al.* (2006).
3 For instance, it is only very recently that gay men's experiences of prostate cancer have begun to receive attention, despite the implications of treatment for gay men's sexual lives and well-being (Filiault *et al.* 2008). Similarly, there has been little consideration of the needs of a growing cohort of older, HIV-positive gay men following the advent of highly active antiretroviral therapies (HAART) in the mid to late 1990s.
4 Barrett's study (2008) also raised the issue of the prescription of Androcur and other androgen suppressants to stifle testosterone and sex drive in those men whose sexuality was perceived to be excessive in the context of institutionalized aged care. The threshold for prescription of Androcur appeared to be lower in situations where staff interpreted gay male clients' sexual behaviour as predatory, raising important questions for further research.

References

Altman, D. (1971) *Homosexual: Oppression and Liberation*, Sydney: Angus & Robertson.
Barrett, C. (2008) *My People: Exploring the Experiences of Gay, Lesbian, Bisexual, Transgender and Intersex Seniors in Aged Care Services*, Melbourne: Matrix Guild Victoria Inc. and Vintage Men Inc.: www.matrixguildvic.org.au (accessed April 2012).

Barrett, C., Harrison, J., and Kent, J. (2009) *Permission to Speak: Towards the Development of Gay, Lesbian, Bisexual, Transgender and Intersex Friendly Aged Care Services*, Melbourne: Matrix Guild Victoria Inc. and Vintage Men Inc.: www.matrixguildvic.org.au (accessed April 2012).

Bauer, M., McAuliffe, L., and Nay, R. (2007) 'Sexuality, health care and the older person: An overview of the literature', *International Journal of Older People Nursing*, 2:63–8.

Bell, D., and Binnie, J. (2000) *The Sexual Citizen: Queer Politics and Beyond*, Cambridge: Polity Press.

Bordo, S. (1999) *The Male Body: A Look at the Male Body in Public and Private*, New York: Farrar, Strauss & Giroux.

Butler, J. (1991) 'Imitation and gender insubordination', in D. Fuss (ed.), *Inside/Out: Lesbian Theories, Gay Theories* (pp. 13–31), London: Routledge.

Cardrona, B. (2008) '"Healthy ageing" policies and anti-ageing ideologies and practices: On the exercise of responsibility', *Medicine, Health Care and Philosophy*, 11: 475–83.

Cole, S. (2000) *Don We Now Our Gay Apparel: Gay Men's Dress in the Twentieth Century*, Oxford: Berg.

Connell, R. W. (2005) *Masculinities*, 2nd edn, Cambridge: Polity Press.

Connell, R. W., and Messerschmidt, J. W. (2005) 'Hegemonic masculinity: Rethinking the concept', *Gender and Society*, 19: 829–59.

Cronin, A., and King, A. (2010) 'Power, inequality and identification: Exploring diversity and intersectionality amongst older LGB adults', *Sociology*, 44: 876–92.

Cummins, D., Trotter, G., Murray, K., Martin, C., and Sutor, A. (2010) 'Development of HIV resource for aged care facilities', *Australian Nurses Journal*, 18: 23.

Didier, E. (2001) 'Michel Foucault's histories of sexuality', *GLQ: A Journal of Lesbian and Gay Studies*, 7(1): 31–86.

Dollimore, J. (1991) *Sexual Dissidence: Augustine to Wilde, Freud to Foucault*, New York: Oxford University Press.

Dowsett, G. W. (1996) *Practicing Desire: Homosexual Sex in the Era of AIDS*, Stanford, CA: Stanford University Press.

Duncan, D. (2009) 'The gay male body: Body image dissatisfaction, identity and reflexive embodiment among gay men', unpublished PhD thesis, Monash University, Melbourne.

Elford, J. (2006) 'Changing patterns of sexual behaviour in the era of highly active antiretorvrial therapy', *Current Opinion in Infectious Diseases*, 19: 26–32.

Ellis, A., and Abarbanel, A. (eds) (1961) *The Encyclopaedia of Sexual Behaviour*, 2 vols, New York: Hawthorn Books.

Faderman, L. (1991) *Odd Girls and Twilight Lovers: A History of Lesbian Life in Twentieth-Century America*, New York: Penguin.

Filiault, S. M., Drummond, M. J., and Smith, J. (2008) 'Gay men and prostate cancer: Voicing the concerns of a hidden population', *Journal of Men's Health and Gender*, 5: 327–32.

Foucault, M. (1988) 'Technologies of the Self', in L. H. Martin, H. Gutman, and P. H. Hatton (eds), *Technologies of the Self* (pp. 16–49), London: Tavistock.

Fredriksen-Goldsen, K., and Muraco, A. (2010) 'Aging and sexual orientation: A 25-year review of the literature', *Research on Aging*, 32: 372–413.

Garber, M. (1992) *Vested Interests: Cross-Dressing and Cultural Anxiety*, London and New York: Penguin Books.

Gardiner, J. (2011) 'Same-sex marriage: A worldwide trend?', in P. Gerber and A. Sifris (eds), *Current Trends in the Regulation of Same-Sex Relationships* (pp. 92–107), special issue, *Law in Context*, 28.

GRAI (GLBTI Retirement Association Inc) and Curtin Health Innovation Research (2010) *Accommodation and Aged Care Issues for Non-Heterosexual Populations*, Perth, Western Australia: GRAI and Curtin Health Innovation Research.

Gregory, A. T., Lowy, M. P., and Zwar, N. A. (2006) 'Men's health and wellbeing: Taking up the challenge in Australia', *Medical Journal of Australia*, 185: 411.

Guasp, A. (2011) *Lesbian, Gay and Bisexual People in Later Life*. London: Stonewall: www.stonewall.org.uk/at_home (accessed April 2012).

Haber, D. (2009) 'Gay aging', *Gerontology and Geriatric Education*, 30: 267–80.

Halkitis, P. N., Zade, D.D., Shrem, M., and Marmor, M. (2004) 'Beliefs about HIV non-infection and risky sexual behaviour among MSM', *AIDS Education and Prevention*, 16: 448–458.

Halperin, D. (1990) *One Hundred Years of Homosexuality and Other Essays on Greek Love*, New York and London: Routledge.

Heaphy, B. (2007) 'Sexualities, gender and ageing: Resources and social change', *Current Sociology*, 55: 193–210.

Heaphy, B., Yip, A. K. T., and Thompson, D. (2004) 'Ageing in a non-heterosexual context', *Ageing and Society*, 24: 881–902.

Hughes, M. (2006) 'Queer ageing', *Gay and Lesbian Issues and Psychology Review*, 2: 54–9.

Jones, J., and Pugh, S. (2005) 'Ageing gay men: Lessons from the sociology of embodiment', *Men and Masculinities*, 7: 248–60.

Katz, S. (2010) 'Sociocultural perspectives on ageing bodies', in D. Dannefer and C. Phillipson (eds), *The Sage Handbook of Social Gerontology* (pp. 557–566), London: Sage.

Katz, S., and Marshall, B. (2003) 'New sex for old: Lifestyle, consumerism, and the ethics of ageing well', *Journal of Ageing Studies*, 17: 3–16.

Kelly, J. (1977) 'The aging homosexual: Myth and reality', *The Gerontologist*, 17: 322–8.

Leonard, W. (2005) 'Queer occupations: Development of Victoria's gay, lesbian, bisexual, transgender and intersex health and wellbeing action plan', *Gay and Lesbian Issues and Psychology Review*, 1: 92–7.

Leonard, W. (in press) 'Safe sex and the aesthetics of gay men's HIV/AIDS prevention in Australia: From *Rubba me* in 1984 to *F**k me* in 2009', *Sexualities*.

Leonard, W., and Mitchell, A. (2000) *The Use of Sexually Explicit Materials in HIV/AIDS Initiatives Targeted at Gay Men: A Guide for Educators*, The Australian National Council on AIDS, Hepatitis C and Related Diseases, Canberra: Commonwealth Department of Health and Aged Care.

Lo, C. (2006) 'We are aged, we are queer, we are here', *Gay and Lesbian Issues and Psychology Review*, 2: 93–7.

National Senior Citizens Law Center (2011) *LGBT Older Adults in Long-Term Care Facilities: Stories from the Field*, publ. by National Senior Citizens Law Center, National Gay and Lesbian Task Force, Services and Advocacy for GLBT Elders (SAGE), Lambda Legal, National Center for Lesbian Rights, National Center for Transgender Equality: www.lgbtlongtermcare.org (accessed April 2012).

Patton, C. (1996) *Fatal Advice: How Safe-Sex Education went Wrong*, Durham, NC, and London: Duke University Press.

Petersen, A. (2007) The *Body in Question: A Socio-Cultural Approach*, London and New York: Routledge.
Potts, A., Grace, V. M., Vares, T., and Gavey, N. (2006) 'Sex for life? Men's counter-stories on "erectile dysfunction", male sexuality and ageing', *Sociology of Health and Illness*, 28: 306–29.
Powell, J. L., Biggs, S., and Wahidan, A. (2006) 'Exploring Foucault and bio-medical gerontology in Western modernity', in J. Powell and A. Wahidin (eds), *Foucault and Ageing* (pp. 3–16), New York: Nova Science Publishers.
Robinson, P. (2008) *The Changing World of Gay Men*, London: Palgrave Macmillan.
Rosenfeld, D. (2010) 'Lesbian, gay, bisexual, and transgender ageing: Shattering myths, capturing lives', in D. Dannefer and C. Phillipson (eds), *The Sage Handbook of Social Gerontology* (pp. 367–376), London: Sage.
Rubin, G. (1984) 'Thinking sex: Notes for a radical theory of the politics of sexuality', in C. Vance (ed.), *Pleasure and Danger: Exploring Female Sexuality* (pp. 276–319), Boston, MA: Routledge & Kegan Paul.
Scherrer, K. S. (2009) 'Images of sexuality and ageing in gerontological literature', *Sexuality Research and Social Policy*, 6: 5–12.
Sedgwick, E. (1990) 'Introduction: Axiomatic', in *Epistemology of the Closet* (pp. 40–59), Berkeley, CA: University of California Press.
Sedgwick, E. (1994) 'How to bring your kids up gay: The war on effeminate boys', in *Tendencies* (pp. 154–166), Durham, NC: Duke University Press.
Sendziuk, P. (2003) *Learning to Trust: Australian Responses to AIDS*, Sydney: UNSW Press.
Simpson, M. (1994) *Male Impersonators: Men Performing Masculinity*, London: Cassell.
Slevin, K. F., and Linneman, T. J. (2010) 'Old gay men's bodies and masculinities', *Men and Masculinities*, 12: 483–507.
Victorian Government Department of Health. (2009) *Well Proud: A Guide to Gay, Lesbian, Bisexual, Transgender and Intersex Inclusive Practice for Health and Human Services*, Melbourne: Ministerial Advisory Committee on Gay, Lesbian, Bisexual, Transgender and Intersex Health and Wellbeing, Victorian Government, Department of Health.
Vincent, J. A. (2009) 'Ageing, anti-ageing, and anti-anti-ageing: Who are the progressives in the debate on the future of human biological ageing?', *Medicine Studies*, 1: 197–208.
Weeks, J. (1985) *Sexuality and its Discontents: Meanings, Myths, and Modern Sexualities*, London: Routledge & Kegan Paul.

Part III
Aging, sexualities and identities

7 Decreasing erectile function and age-appropriate masculinities in Mexico

Emily Wentzell

Jorge's story

I interviewed Jorge, ten years after his testicles were amputated due to cancer, as part of a research project on Mexican men's experiences of changing sexual function. Other participants took similar amputations badly; one feared that he would 'not be a man' after amputation of his penis. However, Jorge appeared to have taken the amputation in stride. A trim man who looked younger than his 82 years, Jorge laughed frequently and spoke with infectious enthusiasm. Jorge was close to his physician, unlike many patients who found it difficult to develop rapport with doctors in their brief and often rigidly hierarchal appointments at the government-run hospital where my research is based. Jorge and his doctor walked into our interview arm-in-arm, the doctor presenting 'Mr. Jorge' as 'an encyclopedia of information' regarding decreased erectile function. While this positive doctor–patient relationship was shaped by both men's unusually upbeat personalities, it was also based on the doctor's respect for Jorge's successful performance of local notions of 'good' older masculinity. The doctor voiced admiration for Jorge's knowledge about life and ability to live happily despite health problems. Rather than feeling robbed of his ability to demonstrate masculinity through penetrative sex, Jorge found fulfillment and earned respect by modelling age-appropriate masculinity.

Jorge's acceptance of decreased later-life erectile function defies both the stereotype of Mexican 'machismo' and the notion, encoded in the medical pathology 'erectile dysfunction' (ED), that 'healthy' men must perform unceasing penetrative sex. In this chapter, I will examine the reasons why, in a site where penetrative sex is often seen as definitive of quintessentially 'Mexican' manhood and where biomedical ED treatments are widely sold and available, older, working-class men overwhelmingly rejected medical interventions for decreased erectile function. I argue that, instead of accepting medicalized understandings of decreased erectile function as ED and seeking pharmaceutical treatment, many men believed frequent sex to be an important but problematic characteristic of youthful manliness that became irrelevant, unbecoming or even dangerous in older age. Using data from interviews with over 250 Mexican male urology patients like Jorge, I will demonstrate that many older men actually understood ED treatment as incompatible with 'good' male aging. I will argue that, in the context of government-funded health care where restricted resources discouraged patients and doctors from medicalizing decreased erectile function, men's widespread rejection of medical treatment for erectile dysfunction was strongly influenced by local ideals of the manly life course.

Jorge described finding happiness in his ability to have 'normal' family relationships, which he stressed were different from the 'macho' interactions that he said stereotypically characterized Mexican men's family interactions. As I will discuss in depth later, machismo is a form of Mexican masculinity marked by sexual rapaciousness, emotional closure, violence and womanizing that Mexicans both widely critique and frequently identify in their own culture (McKee Irwin 2003). Jorge said that his testicular cancer diagnosis made him very concerned about his health, but not about the fact that life-saving surgery would end his ability to have penetrative sex. He reported that the surgery did not bother him 'as a man' because 'I really thought it was necessary – it didn't cause me much stress. I keep moving forward. I didn't feel that it took away my masculinity.' Jorge explained that he disagreed with the idea that a man who could not have sex was unmanly, believing that it was more important for a man to be healthy than to have sex. He said, 'I preferred to lose them [his testicles] than to develop the cancer. They told me it was one or the other.'

A key reason why Jorge was unconcerned by surgically induced erectile function change was because it did not disrupt his expected manly life course. Jorge believed that a 'normal' man's life involved decreasing emphasis on penetrative sexuality over time, as his had even before his amputation. Jorge said he began to experience decreasing erectile function in his late 50s, and understood it as a 'natural' aspect of aging. He contextualized this change within changing family relationships over time, stating, 'I had erection problems from age 58. I was married almost 45 years; we had five children, my wife died on me twelve years ago. In 1996, I was left a widower.' Jorge thus understood cessation of erectile function as part of a culturally intelligible and 'normal' life-course narrative. He valued adherence to this normal course of male aging, in which one marries, has children and ages with a spouse, rather than the unceasing penetrative sexuality that he associated with 'macho' Mexican masculinity.

Thus, Jorge did not see his decreasing erectile function as 'unnatural' or a medical concern. When I asked why he thought it occurred, he explained that it was not because of illness, but 'Because of my nature. I never sought a medical solution to this problem – I just thought that my sex life was ending.' Jorge reported that, after age 58, he and his wife had sex occasionally, 'but it wasn't even something I sought out'. He said, 'In our married life, we were very happy. When the sex life ended, ok, we knew it would end one day. So, there wasn't treatment – I never tried anything. I really didn't have a problem with it.' Jorge did not see testicular amputation as an impediment to being a normal man, since he sought to enact 'good' masculinity through age-appropriate relationships rather than sexual prowess.

Jorge simply did not see his capacity to have penetrative sex as relevant to his ability to be a good older man. He said he felt satisfied by strong relationships with family members and his active participation in his grown children's lives, like living with and assisting an unmarried daughter. He also had a successful romantic relationship despite his inability to have penetrative sex. For two years, he had been dating a widow in her mid-70s, with whom he spent leisure time and travelled. This relationship was important to his sense of well-being. He explained, 'It's very important to love someone, to have someone to love you.' He did not see lack of penetrative sex as an impediment to love, explaining that his girlfriend would 'like to have sex, but I can't – medications are dangerous for me, I have heart problems. She'd like me to have erections, but since I know there won't be any, I don't miss it.' Jorge instead sought satisfaction 'as a man' through a caring relationship with a partner who accepted the consequences of his testicular amputation, rather than seeking to regain erectile function and live out a masculinity focused on penetrative sex.

Erectile dysfunction, global discourse and local difference

Less-than-ideal erections have been understood differently across time and place, from a natural result of aging, to a symptom of stress, to a result of witchcraft (Wentzell 2008; McLaren 2007). Since the 1998 introduction of Viagra, a drug which facilitates penile erection, a global 'medicalization of impotence' has occurred in which erectile difficulty is diagnosed as the biomedical pathology 'erectile dysfunction' (ED) (Tiefer 1994). ED is now widely diagnosed and treated; annual global ED drug sales average around $2.5 billion (Berenson 2006). This medicalization of erectile function change entails pathologization of variation in men's sexual function. The medical definition of erectile dysfunction as 'the inability to attain or maintain penile erection sufficient for satisfactory sexual intercourse' obscures the fact that definitions of 'sufficient' erection and 'satisfactory' sex reflect cultural standards that link ideal masculinity to penetrative sexuality (Lizza and Rosen 1999: 141; Tiefer 2006). ED drugs may thus function as 'masculinity pills' (Loe 2006: 31). By providing a biological 'cure' for failing masculinity that obscures the social context of sexuality, these drugs naturalize Western notions of male sexuality as mechanistic, unflagging and asocial (Grace *et al.* 2006; Mamo and Fishman 2001). The concept of ED also pathologizes sexual changes related to aging (Marshall and Katz 2002). ED drugs encode a narrow definition of 'healthy' male sexuality: that men of any age and health status should want and achieve erections that enable frequent penetrative sex.

Despite the globalization of this homogenizing notion, people relate to drugs like Viagra in locally specific ways. Use of globally sold pharmaceuticals varies according to structural and cultural context, including local gender ideals and understandings of health (Petryna *et al.* 2006; van der Geest *et al.* 1996). While ED drugs are designed to facilitate mechanistic manly sexuality, they may be used to enact varying performances of masculinity, broadly defined as 'what men say and do *to be men*' (Gutmann 1996: 17; emphasis his). Varying national discourses on masculinity and ED drugs, including government drug approval practices and debates about the social role of biomedicine, also shape individuals' decisions about ED drugs' appropriateness (Castro-Vásquez 2006; Sugishita 2009). Thus, individuals relate to multiple discourses, and are influenced by multiple structural factors, as they decide how to regard diminishing erections.

In Mexico, ED drugs have been popular sellers and discussion topics since Viagra's introduction. ED pharmaceuticals and herbal copycats like 'Powersex' and 'Himcaps' are widely advertised, and the label 'Viagra' is often attached to ostensible aphrodisiacs, like sea urchin 'Viagra' soup. ED is a common punch line in jokes on TV and between friends. Based on this popularity and the fact that ED drugs facilitate the sort of frequent sexual penetration definitive of 'machismo', it would seem that Mexican men as a group would welcome ED drugs. However, my research revealed that older, working-class, urban Mexican men like Jorge overwhelmingly rejected the notion that decreasing erectile function in later life was a medical pathology, characterizing ED drug treatment as unnecessary or even deadly. After describing this research, I will analyse the ways that local understandings of health, masculinity and the ideal manly life course, together with economic disincentives for medicalizing decreased erectile function, shaped older, working-class Mexican men's rationales for rejecting ED drugs.

Study methods and ethics

This chapter is based on findings from an ethnographic study of men's experiences of aging, illness and changing sexual function in the central Mexican city of Cuernavaca in 2007–8. This research was based in the urology department of a hospital in the federal Instituto Méxicano del Seguro Social (IMSS) system, which offers care to all privately employed workers and their dependants (about half of the Mexican population) (INEGI 2005). Due to long waiting times and sometimes scarce resources at IMSS facilities, eligible patients who can afford private care often opt out. Thus, most men I interviewed were working class. While they or a close relative held formal employment and thus had some amount of steady income, most lacked the economic resources to pay for private health care. As I will discuss in the next section, this scarcity of resources for medical treatment discouraged both these men and their IMSS physicians from understanding sometimes-medicalized bodily changes like erectile difficulty as medical problems.

My research centred on semi-structured Spanish-language ethnographic interviews with 250 male IMSS urology patients. All had either experienced decreasing erectile function due to aging or illness, or had received a diagnosis that suggested that this bodily change was imminent. The data presented in this chapter are thus drawn from participants with varying degrees of erectile difficulty, experiencing illnesses of varying severity (from life-threatening cancer to well-controlled heart disease). In our conversations, I aimed to discover how men understood their experiences of bodily change, especially age- and illness-related changes in sexual function, to have shaped their ideas about and practices of masculinity. In semi-structured interviews, participants discussed their health histories, romantic lives, families and work experiences. Avoiding abstract questions about 'masculinity', I asked concrete questions about individuals' life and health experiences and understandings of what made one a 'good' or 'bad' husband, father and sexual partner. I interviewed about 50 of these participants together with their wives, revealing the ways that they negotiated and jointly assigned meaning to the experiences of sexual change and medical treatment.

I interviewed men ranging in age from their late teens to their 90s. However, since most participants were seeking treatment for age-related prostate problems or urologic symptoms of chronic illnesses like type-2 diabetes, most study participants were in their 50s–60s. Since aging is central to the present analysis, it is important to note that participants tended to describe themselves or others as 'older' versus 'younger', not based on numeric age, but on whether they were performing behaviours more culturally associated with youthful or more 'mature' masculinity. For instance, while participants commonly saw themselves as 'older' beginning in their 50s or 60s, some did not consider themselves 'older' until the onset of chronic illness in their 80s or 90s. While for purposes of clarity I will gloss certain ideals of masculinity as belonging to 'older' men, this categorization refers to participants' self-definitions rather than numeric ages. While these 'older' men often shared the views on socially appropriate male aging and Mexican masculinity discussed below, their experiences and ideas were by no means homogeneous.

Finally, despite the stereotype that Mexican men might not discuss sexual difficulty with women, men asked to participate were very enthusiastic, with about 96 percent of patients approached participating. My positionality as a female, American researcher facilitated their participation and openness, since many participants said they felt comfortable telling a woman things they felt ashamed to tell another man. Many also said they assumed that American women were sexually knowledgeable, so they felt able to say things they feared would shock a Mexican woman. Our different genders, ages and nationalities surely shaped the kinds of things study participants told me and ways they framed their experiences. Rather than generating journalistic accounts of men's health and sexual practices, our interactions generated narratives regarding men's experiences that they characterized as 'confessional'. Participants frequently reported enjoying 'the chance to talk' about sexual and health issues that they often felt unable to discuss with peers or partners. While partial, these narratives thus provided key insights into the links men drew between their erectile function change, medical experience and ways of 'being men'. Since such openness was based on my assurance of confidentiality, all names given here are pseudonyms.

Understandings of health, aging and ED drugs in Mexico and the IMSS

Although biomedicine is the most widely used healing system in Mexico, Mexican biomedical practices are influenced by other locally important ways of understanding health. Obviously, as IMSS patients, study participants had faith in biomedicine as a valid way to understand bodily distress and to treat physical ailments. Yet for most, biomedical perspectives were one of many belief systems they used to make sense of health and illness. Many Mexicans hold hybrid understandings of bodies and health, combining biomedical understandings of sickness with the ideas that psychological and emotional trouble are inseparable from bodily distress, and that a lack of bodily or emotional 'balance' can also cause illness (Congress 1992; Finkler 1991). Study participants relied on a combination of these three ways of understanding health and the body when discussing the causes and courses of their illnesses and bodily changes.

Most participants believed that strong negative emotions could cause physical ailments. Throughout Latin America and its diaspora, people identify emotional conditions like *susto* (fright), *nervios* (nerves) and *coraje* (rage) as 'illnesses of emotion' that trigger a range of physical pathologies (Rubel *et al.* 1985; Baer *et al.* 2003; Guarnaccia *et al.* 1996; Finkler 1991). Many participants described the ways in which negative emotion created physical symptoms. For instance, a 45 year-old gardener said that worrying about the deterioration of his marriage had caused bodily damage, giving him 'stress and nerves (*nervios*)'; he emphasized that 'nerves are physical'. Participants often said that strong emotions increased their vulnerability to biomedical diseases. For instance, the wife of a 62-year-old retired salesman said his diabetes onset was caused by a 'very strong rage (*coraje*) over family problems'. As these examples of illness caused by familial strife show, illnesses of emotion can relate to gender in that the strong negative feelings that cause them often relate to people's difficulties in being 'good' husbands, wives and parents (Rebhun 1993; Finkler 1994).

Some participants also subscribed to 'humoral', or balance-related, notions of bodily health and function. Throughout Latin America and other world regions, people ascribe properties of literal or metaphorical 'hotness' or 'coldness' to illnesses, injuries, activities, remedies and personality traits, believing that excesses or inappropriate mixes of even metaphorical cold or heat can do concrete physical damage (Foster 1994). Participants frequently said that very hot or cold weather exacerbated chronic illnesses like diabetes, making it difficult to work or increasing symptoms like thirst or swelling.

Decreasing erectile function and age-appropriate masculinities 129

Some believed that extreme hot or cold weather itself caused bodily harm, like the 55-year-old gardener who said that more than thirty years of working outside in the early morning had made him permanently 'cold', causing chills and urinary problems. He had come to the doctor because, 'I wanted something to warm my body.' Conversely, participants occasionally stated that their overly 'hot' constitutions, expressed through frequent sex in their youths, had done damage that resulted in currently decreasing erectile function.

Overall, study participants generally saw illnesses as biomedically treatable, but explicable only through simultaneous attention to emotional disturbance and disruption of bodily balance. In keeping with this relational understanding of health, in which social, behavioural and emotional context are crucial components of the disease processes, participants frequently voiced the expectation that their bodies would change over time. Mexican users of biomedicine thus understood socially appropriate relationships between bodily function, behaviour and social context as key sources of the balance and emotional calm necessary for good health. In this context, participants' ideas about what constituted 'healthy' sexual behaviour were intimately related to their beliefs about age-appropriate behaviour and embodiment. Participants frequently said that since aging bodies naturally 'slowed', vigorous activity, including frequent sex, might do physical harm in older age. Instead of seeing the ability to perform unceasing, mechanistic penetrative sex despite age or illness, as a sign of health, most older participants saw Viagra-mediated sexuality as age-inappropriate, unbalancing and thus a potential cause of illness.

These beliefs led the vast majority of older study participants who had experienced decreasing erectile function to reject ED treatment. While all were familiar with drugs like Viagra, most did not see them as necessary for a change that was, as Jorge articulated, 'natural'. Participants often characterized diminished sexual frequency as 'part of the process', and, as an 82-year-old retired accountant described, 'something that I've lived. It's nature, I'm diminishing, and I take that as something normal.' They thus rejected ED drugs because, as a 56-year-old machinery operator stated, 'I don't like to use things that aren't normal. I don't like to force my body.' In fact, they believed that by forcing vulnerable, aging bodies to perform unnatural behaviour, ED drugs could do serious harm.

Rather than seeing ED drugs as solving the problem of decreasing erectile function, these participants believed that they would cause a physical problem, by forcing the embodiment of inappropriately 'youthful' sexuality in older age. Many feared that thwarting natural changes through medical intervention might dangerously 'accelerate' one's body at a time when it was naturally slowing down. For example, a 78-year-old food vendor explained that he and his peers believed that ED drugs were dangerous because they 'accelerate you, to your death. Many friends have told me, they will accelerate you a lot, then you'll collapse, that stuff will kill you.' Several other participants recounted rumours of deaths caused when elderly men had foolishly taken ED drugs. While some older men were wistful about the frequent sexuality they had enjoyed in their younger days, even those who wished to continue some form of sex tended to reject drugs like Viagra. Instead, they tended to take vitamins or try to improve their diet or exercise habits, seeing these actions as gentler alternatives that could facilitate erection by improving their general health, but would not dangerously disrupt or unbalance their natural process of bodily aging (Wentzell and Salmerón 2009).

Structural factors including individuals' incomes and the nature of IMSS medical appointments also contributed to this phenomenon. The IMSS system is legally required to dispense a set list of drugs, which included an ED medication, cost-free to any patients who are prescribed them. However, the lack of resources at the Cuernavaca IMSS hospital meant that in practice its pharmacy did not stock this ED drug. Although participants did not usually mention drug prices as a reason that they did not seek ED treatment, the cost of having to purchase the drugs privately surely provided an additional disincentive for understanding decreased erectile function as a medical problem. Several IMSS urologists also told me that they rarely prescribed ED drugs to their patients partly because many of the men were older, but also in part because the prescriptions could not be filled at the hospital (in contrast, they reported prescribing ED drugs much more commonly in their private practices). In addition to the discouragement from diagnosing ED posed by the IMSS pharmacy's failure to provide ED drugs, the rushed and often impersonal nature of appointments at the overscheduled IMSS hospital created an atmosphere that was not conducive to discussion of sexual difficulty. Doctors were likely to use appointment time to address only a patient's most life-threatening conditions, while many participants reported to me that they did not feel that they had time to develop enough trust with their doctors to discuss sex. These structural factors likely compounded older, working-class IMSS patients' culturally based aversion to drug treatment for decreasing erectile function.

'Machismo' and problematic youthful sexuality

Despite the global marketing of ED treatments that equate unceasing virility with health, participants understood a 'natural' and age-appropriate slowing of sexuality to be healthy. Their commonly held idea that frequent, penetrative sexuality is physically inappropriate for older men was supported by their often-stated belief that 'macho' sexuality was natural to Mexican men, but socially negative. For this reason, men often understood age-related bodily changes that slowed down one's sex life to enable positive behavioural changes.

Individuals, politicians and the Mexican media frequently discuss the necessity – and difficulty – of embracing 'modern', or more egalitarian, gender roles (Szasz 1998a; Amuchástegui and Szasz 2007). In Mexico as in many other world regions, companionate marriage, focused on emotional closeness rather than, or in addition to, the economic production and social reproduction central to traditional forms of marriage, has become the ideal, and is seen as an appropriately 'modern' form of interpersonal interaction (Carillo 2007; Hirsch 2003; Wardlow and Hirsch 2006). Yet while most study participants defined such 'modern' marital relationships as ideal, they also consistently described Mexican men's 'macho' nature – especially when expressed through the frequent extramarital sex made possible by youthful, healthful bodies – as a barrier to achieving close or faithful relationships.

Machismo is a patriarchal style of masculinity, characterized by high sexual desire, womanizing and emotional withdrawal. This understanding of Mexican manliness is actually quite recent, popularized by poet and cultural commentator Octavio Paz in the 1950s (Paz 1985). Paz asserted that Mexican men were inherently remote, emotionally unyielding and sexually aggressive because of their historic status as *hijos de la chingada*, or sons of indigenous women raped by conquistadors (1985: 75). Paz argued that, as the product of these coercive unions, Mexican men were predisposed to enact intimate violence in an endless quest to play the role of conqueror rather than conquered. While Paz's work was a literary interpretation of Mexican history and society rather than a social scientific account of the lived reality of gender in the nation, his characterization of machismo has been immensely influential, becoming a central, if widely contested, way that Mexicans define 'the Mexican man's' innate tendencies (Gutmann 1996; McKee Irwin 2003; Ramirez 2009; Szasz 1998b).

While I never broached the term 'machismo' in interviews, almost all study participants referenced it as an aspect of Mexican masculinity that, for better or worse, had shaped their own ways of being men, especially in their youths. Some participants said they had tried to act against machismo, while others used the concept to explain their past behaviours. Despite this diversity, most participants characterized the abstract 'Mexican man' as intrinsically and problematically macho. Participants frequently biologized machismo, explaining that the 'hot' Mexican constitution predisposed men to want frequent sex with a variety of women, overindulge in alcohol and carouse. For example, a 56-year-old veterinarian told me that, 'Here in Mexico, [infidelity is] something normal. They say the Mexican is passionate. They say the man is polygamous by nature.' Other participants followed Paz's logic, telling me that machismo was a cultural inheritance from the founding of their nation and before. For example, a 24-year-old gym teacher saw machismo as a historical response to men's ongoing fears of losing control of relationships with women. He said, 'A lot of machismo exists ... They're afraid that if they let their guard down, they'll become whipped. That's the closed psychology of the macho man, from prehispanic times.' Whether they saw machismo as cultural or biological, participants believed that men with bodies young and healthy enough to have frequent extramarital sex would be predisposed to do so.

Yet even those men who described living out machismo while they were physically able understood this style of masculinity to be socially problematic. A 58-year-old driver told me that Mexican men are taught that 'the woman needs to be behind', but that they must learn that 'The wife isn't a thing – she's a person, she's a comrade.' Similarly, a 51-year-old librarian critiqued the fact that 'Here in Mexico, it's seen as bad if a man does the housework – they call him whipped', stating that since women were now working outside the home and the nation was changing, 'men are going to have to change their attitude'. Through such language, participants often described Mexican society as undergoing a slow movement away from macho masculinity, which they saw reflected in their own lives as they were prompted by changing bodies to age out of frequent, extramarital sexuality. Conversely, some older and most of the smaller group of younger men I interviewed called for lifelong rejection of machismo, often saying they tried to live out more modern and positive forms of masculinity by 'being different than my father' (for discussion of use of ED drugs to assert generational difference, see Wentzell 2011). In the context of their beliefs that machismo was both innate to the abstract 'Mexican man' and a problematic barrier to national advancement, study participants looked unfavourably on pharmaceutical interventions that facilitated macho sexuality.

Ideals of changing sexuality across the male life course

Around the world, beliefs about whether or how men's sexual activity should change as they age reflect the intersection of medicalized understandings of erectile difficulty and other age-related changes with local cultural understandings about what constitutes 'good' behaviour for older men (for a discussion of the ways some Turkish men relate to the medical discourse of 'andropause,' see Erol and Özbay, this volume). For example, older men in Ghana are expected to embody respectability by focusing more on family and less on sex as they age (van der Geest 2001), while men in North America and Western Europe often seek respect by appearing physically and sexually 'youthful' for as long as possible (Loe 2004; Marshall and Katz 2002; Sandberg 2007).

In Mexico, beliefs about machismo's naturalness and social dangerousness powerfully influence men's beliefs about how one should be sexual and respectable in older age. Whether study participants rejected machismo or identified it as driving some of their own behaviours, the vast majority of men I interviewed shared the belief that the frequent sex associated with machismo was radically inappropriate for older men. Thus, in contrast to the valorization of unchanging sexual frequency central to the biomedical concept of ED, study participants thought that the kind of sex a man had should ideally change over the course of his life. Rather than viewing continued penetrative sex as definitive of successful manliness across the life course, many participants said that they sought to embody 'respectable' and age-appropriate older manhood by moving away from machismo, changing their sexual practices and relationships as they aged.

Most participants told me that the macho sexuality that they saw as age-appropriate, if socially problematic, for younger men seemed frankly absurd to them in older age. In response to a question about whether he would continue to seek extramarital sex, a 68-year-old barber laughed and said, 'Here in Mexico, we have a saying: "In old age, chickenpox" ... it means that some things become silly when one is older.' This absurdity stemmed from the idea that 'good' older masculinity entailed a shift of focus from the outside world to one's family, especially in terms of giving up extramarital sex in favour of a focus on one's family's feelings. Many participants believed that older men's lives should become domestically oriented. Participants said that, as older men, they felt duty-bound to provide emotional support and family leadership – for instance, by being a 'role model' for grandchildren – which they had not previously seen as important to being 'good' men. Typifying this expected life change, a 56-year-old stated that after his retirement from the public health service, 'I will dedicate myself to my wife, the house, gardening, caring for the grandchildren – the Mexican classic.' The majority of older participants reported that different behaviours made them feel 'like men' at different times; these practices included having frequent extramarital sex when younger, and curtailing such behaviour in order to focus on their homes and families as they aged.

In the context of this shared ideal of changing masculinity over time, most participants reported initial dismay at the experience of decreased erectile function, but said they had come to accept it because it actually facilitated their shift to age-appropriate older masculinity. For example, many came to understand erectile function change as a clear bodily signal that their youth had ended and it was time to start behaving differently. Further, many reported that the embodied experience of decreased erectile function enabled them to pursue new and differently fulfilling forms of sexuality and marriage.

For example, as their erectile function waned, many participants began to increasingly incorporate companionate ideals for marriage, which had not figured in some older men's youthful decisions about marriage and family, into their own relationships. They did so partly because these notions of marriage had become culturally dominant, and partly because the idea that husbands and wives should be emotionally close fit well with their expected later-life shift of emphasis to home and family. Many older participants told me that, as they ceased to focus so much on work and affairs, they forged more emotionally intimate and often very rewarding relationships with their families. Some stated that this was partly enabled by the diminishment of bodily urges for sex that accompanied aging. For example, a 77-year-old retiree explained that sexual passion 'is like a flower. It has a beautiful moment, but fades with the passage of time.' He told me that 'sexual love' for one's wife changes over time into a deeper form of affection that is 'less based on sexual contact'. Thus, older participants tended to discuss frequent, penetrative sex as a pleasurable but socially problematic practice that was important to younger but not older men's lives. A 75-year-old retired factory worker succinctly stated, 'Erectile dysfunction isn't important. When I was young, it would have been, but not now.' Similarly, a 64-year-old retired mechanic stated that his, 'Sex life now doesn't exist, doesn't exist. But, I'm satisfied, from my youth. I don't miss it.' Participants' general rejection of ED drugs makes sense in this context where decreasing erectile function actually paves the way for new and 'respectable' forms of emotional fulfillment.

Stereotypic masculinities and local complexities

On the surface, ED drugs' popularity in Mexico seems over-determined. Mexicans use biomedicine more than any other healing system, and from a biomedical perspective, decreased erectile function is a physical pathology. The ability to medicate away erectile difficulty also seems to resonate with the 'macho' form of sex-obsessed masculinity that is so commonly attributed to 'the Mexican man', even by the Mexican study participants themselves. And indeed, drugs like Viagra are popular, both as a topic of conversation and as a pharmaceutical intervention, in Mexico. However, the older, working-class men in my study population were highly unlikely to use ED treatment. Less than 4 percent of these study participants, mostly men who reported still feeling 'young', tried drugs like Viagra (see Wentzell and Salmerón 2009). Other Mexican populations, especially wealthier men receiving treatment for health problems similar to those experienced by study participants from private physicians, and well as younger men seeking sexual enhancement in keeping with the sexual ideals of 'machismo', are far more likely to use ED drugs (Wentzell 2009).

This demographic difference in men's likelihood of desiring or using ED treatment reveals an important exception to the stereotypic assumption that Mexican men in general would be a prime ED drug market. The confluence of local debates about negative consequences of 'machismo', health beliefs that made pharmaceutical sexual enhancement seem dangerous for older bodies, and understandings of the manly life course that made 'youthful' sexuality seem radically inappropriate in older age, led older study participants to see ED drugs as absurd and possibly harmful. Like the ideas that shape it, their rejection of erection-enhancing pharmaceuticals is context-dependent. It is likely that older men's common view of the life course as ideally shifting from a more macho to a domestic orientation will be outmoded when today's younger men, who often seek to engage in companionate marriage from the start, begin to grow old. Members of this next generation, who frequently view emotion-laden sex as a key element of a happy marriage, might use ED drugs to avoid changes in sexuality that might threaten their relationships. Similarly, as biomedical understandings of health and bodies gain increasing global dominance, subsequent generations of men may not temper biomedical understandings of sexual function with ideas about the importance of balance and calm emotion for health.

Overall, the non-generalizablity of older, working-class Mexican men's understandings of sexuality, masculinity and health demonstrates the importance of attending to place, time and context when investigating men's experiences of aging and health. Participants' rejection of ED drugs, even as they accepted biomedical treatment for other ailments, shows that the presence of medicalized models of experience does not necessarily mean that people will adopt them uncritically. Structural conditions in the IMSS system, including rushed appointments and economic barriers to cost-free access to ED drugs, encourage people to interpret bodily changes as natural or pathological in ways that link cultural norms and the financial feasibility of receiving medical treatment. Participants' views present a reminder that biomedicine is a cultural system, used in contexts where definitions of a healthy sex life are shaped by local ideals about gender, aging, sex and love. Thus, despite the globally-marketed biomedical messages about healthy male sexuality and the widespread stereotype of Mexican machismo, men like Jorge are able to reject these models for manhood, asserting 'good' masculinity by embracing what others might consider 'erectile dysfunction'.

References

Amuchástegui, A., and Szasz, I. (eds) (2007) *Sucede que me canso de ser hombre*, Mexico City: El Colegio de Mexico.
Baer, R. D., Weller, S. C., Garcia de Alba Garcia, J., Glazer, M., Trotter, R., Pachter, L., and Klein, R. E. (2003) 'A cross-cultural approach to the study of the folk illness nervios', *Culture, Medicine and Psychiatry*, 27: 315–37.
Berenson, A. (2006) 'A daily pill to combat impotence?', *New York Times* (13 June).
Carillo, H. (2007) 'Imagining modernity: Sexuality, policy, and social change in Mexico', *Sexuality Research and Social Policy: Journal of NSRC*, 4: 74–91.
Castro-Vásquez, G. (2006) 'The politics of Viagra: Gender, dysfunction and reproduction in Japan', *Body and Society*, 12: 109–29.
Congress, E. P. (1992) 'Cultural differences in health beliefs: Implications for social work practice in health care settings', *Social Work in Health Care*, 17: 81–96.
Finkler, K. (1991) *Physicians at Work, Patients in Pain: Biomedical Practice and Patient Response in Mexico*, Boulder, CO: Westview Press.
Finkler, K. (1994) *Women in Pain: Gender and Morbidity in Mexico*, Philadelphia, PA: University of Pennslyania Press.
Foster, G. M. (1994) *Hippocrates' Latin American Legacy: Humoral Medicine in the New World*, Langhorne, PA: Gordon & Breach.
Grace, V., Potts, A., Gavey, N., and Vares, T. (2006) 'The discursive condition of Viagra', *Sexualities*, 9: 295–314.
Guarnaccia, P. J., Rivera, M., Franco, F., and Neighbors, C. (1996) 'The experiences of ataques de nervios: Towards an anthropology of emotions in Puerto Rico', *Culture, Medicine and Psychiatry*, 20: 343–67.
Gutmann, M. C. (1996) *The Meanings of Macho: Being a Man in Mexico City*, Berkeley, CA: University of California Press.

Hirsch, J. (2003) *A Courtship After Marriage: Sexuality and Love in Mexican Transnational Families*, Berkeley, CA: University of California Press.

INEGI (2005) 'Causas seleccionadas de mortalidad por sexo 2005', in *Estadísticas vitales 2005*, Mexico City: INEGI.

Lizza, E., and Rosen, R. (1999) 'Definition and classification of erectile dysfunction: Report of the Nomenclature Committee of the International Society of Impotence Research', *International Journal of Impotence Research*, 11: 141–3.

Loe, M. (2004) *The Rise of Viagra: How the Little Blue Pill Changed Sex in America*, New York: New York University Press.

Loe, M. (2006) 'The Viagra blues: Embracing or resisting the Viagra body', in D. Rosenfeld and C. A. Faircloth (eds), *Medicalized Masculinities* (pp. 315–332), Philadelphia, PA: Temple University Press.

McKee Irwin, R. (2003) *Mexican Masculinities*, Minneapolis, MN: University of Minnesota Press.

McLaren, A. (2007) *Impotence: A Cultural History*, Chicago, IL: University of Chicago Press.

Mamo, L., and Fishman, J. (2001) 'Potency in all the right places: Viagra as a technology of the gendered body', *Body and Society*, 7: 13–35.

Marshall, B. L., and Katz, S. (2002) 'Forever functional: Sexual fitness and the ageing male body', *Body and Society*, 8: 43–70.

Paz, O. (1985) *The Labyrinth of Solitude and Other Writings*, New York: Grove Weidenfeld (orig. 1961).

Petryna, A., Lakoff, A., and Kleinman, A. (eds) (2006) *Global Pharmaceuticals: Ethics, Markets, Practices*, Durham, NC: Duke University Press.

Ramirez, J. (2009) *Against Machismo: Young Adult Voices in Mexico City*, New York: Berghahn Books.

Rebhun, L. A. (1993) 'Nerves and emotional play in northeast Brazil', *Medical Anthropology Quarterly*, 7: 131–51.

Rubel, A. J., O'Nell, C. W., and Collado-Ardón, R. (1985) *Susto: A Folk Illness*, Berkeley, CA: University of California Press.

Sandberg, L. (2007) 'Ancient monuments, mature men and those popping amphetamine: Researching the lives of older men', *Nordic Journal for Masculinity Studies*, 2: 85–108.

Sugishita, K. (2009) 'Traditional medicine, biomedicine and Christianity in modern Zambia', *Africa: The Journal of the International African Institute*, 79: 435–54.

Szasz, I. (1998a) 'Los hombres y la sexualidad: Aportes desde la perspectiva feminista y primeros acercamientos a su estudio en México', in S. Lerner (ed.), *Varones, sexualidad y reproducción: Diversas perspectivas teórico-metodológicas y hallazgos de investigación* (pp. 137–162), Mexico City: El Colegio de México/Somede.

Szasz, I. (1998b) 'Masculine identity and the meanings of sexuality: A review of research in Mexico', *Reproductive Health Matters*, 6: 97–104.

Tiefer, L. (1994) 'The medicalization of impotence: Normalizing phallocentrism', *Gender and Society*, 8: 363–77.

Tiefer, L. (2006) 'The Viagra phenomenon', *Sexualities*, 9: 273–94.

van der Geest, S. (2001) '"No strength": Sex and old age in a rural town in Ghana', *Social Science and Medicine*, 53: 1383–96.

van der Geest, S., Whyte, S. R., and Hardon, A. (1996) 'The anthropology of pharmaceuticals: A biographical approach', *Annual Review of Anthropology*, 25: 153–78.

Wardlow, H., and Hirsch, J. S. (2006) 'Introduction', in J. S. Hirsch and H. Wardlow (eds), *Modern Loves: The Anthropology of Romantic Courtship and Companionate Marriage* (pp. 1–31), Ann Arbor: University of Michigan Press.

Wentzell, E. (2008) 'Imagining impotence in America: From men's deeds to men's minds to Viagra', *Michigan Discussions in Anthropology*, 25: 153–78.

Wentzell, E. (2009) 'Composite masculinities: Aging, illness, erectile dysfunction and Mexican manhood', PhD, University of Michigan.

Wentzell, E. (2011) 'Generational differences in Mexican men's ideas of age-appropriate sex and Viagra use', *Men and Masculinities*, 14: 392–407.

Wentzell, E., and Salmerón, J. (2009) 'You'll "get Viagraed": Mexican men's preference for alternative erectile dysfunction treatment', *Social Science and Medicine*, 68: 1759–65.

8 Enhancing masculinity and sexuality in later life through modern medicine

Experiences of polygynous Yoruba men in southwest Nigeria

Agunbiade Ojo Melvin

Introduction

Sexuality across the life course mirrors the values, norms and judgments of the society (Bauer *et al.* 2007). Each culture has a gendered lens, presenting multiple notions of what is masculine and feminine (Rosaldo and Lamphere 1974). As social actors, we aspire to imitate the societal image of being a male or female, which often creates contradictions and pressures (West and Zimmerman 1987; Butler 1990). Thus, masculinity entails an engagement with practices or acts available within a given cultural context, often producing dominance of one form or another. However, the notion of masculinity changes according to context and life events, especially in later life (Bennett 2007). With critical insights from the literature (Kampf and Botelho 2009; Vincent 2006) and attention to the dynamics of masculinity and sexuality in later life, this chapter undertakes a cultural interpretation of anti-aging medicine; and how men approach bodily changes and their sexuality. With an increasing wave of anti-aging medicine supported by an emerging global consumer culture, it presents a cultural interrogation of everyday practices that involve the use of modern medicine in heterosexual relations. With an initial focus on polygyny as a form of marriage shaped by notions of dominant masculinity, the chapter further examines the cultural beliefs influencing men's acts and practices in relation to medicine use. Empirical evidence was generated through face-to-face in-depth interviews with polygynous Yoruba men, exploring their engagement with cultural constructions of masculinity, aging and sexuality. Interviews were also conducted with modern health caregivers.

Polygyny and masculinities

Polygyny is a common practice in many African societies. It refers to a form of marriage in which men have multiple wives (co-wives), as opposed to polyandrous polygamy, in which a woman has multiple husbands (Falen

2008). In African society, most women in polygynous marriage are younger in age than their husbands. This may be associated with the high premium placed on fertility within marriage (Hollos *et al.* 2009). Based on the asymmetrical power relations, Bove and Valeggia (2009) describe polygyny as 'co-operative conflicts within households'. Within this social arrangement, the notions of masculinity and femininity are often invoked in addressing tensions and strains, including those associated with sexual relations.

In many African cultures, heterosexuality and masculinity have been dominant forms of sexual expressions throughout the life course, while other forms of sexualities have been marginalized (Tamale 2011). Most studies dealing with masculinity and sexuality among older men (see e.g. Alex *et al.* 2008; Calasanti 2004; Thompson 1994) are from developed countries. While some studies have focused on health issues among middle-aged and older populations in Nigeria, their aims are restricted to health challenges, especially chronic and acute conditions (Bekibele and Gureje 2010; Adebusoye *et al.* 2011). A number of Nigerian studies that have examined the influence of masculinity on sexual practices focused on HIV among youths and adolescents (Asuquo 1999; Izugbara 2001; Olawoye *et al.* 2004). No known Nigerian study has explored the practices and experiences of middle-aged and older polygynous men in enhancing their sexualities within heterosexual relationships, despite the historical and cultural presence of polygynous marriages (Igenoza 2007).

Positions that emphasize beliefs and medicine use among older adults only in relation to acute and chronic health conditions may be over-representing biomedical positions on aging to the neglect of experiences of aging from the actors' perspective. Aging is a multi-dimensional reality with both objective and subjective consequences for the individual and the society. While the use of sexuopharmaceutical drugs is on the increase (Loe 2004), African studies focusing on the experiences of middle-aged and older men who use such drugs to remain sexually active are scarce. Attention to this issue is important if we are to address concerns such as those of Willison and Andrews (2004) who decried the lack of critical gerontological perspectives on the cultural determinants of medicine use among older people, and the absence of studies exploring the subjective experiences of older people.

Sexuality in a historical and cultural context is shrouded by different ethical expectations and rights explorations (Foucault 1990; Weeks 2003). In ethical terms, the consequences for individuals of conforming to the various contradictions and pressures within cultural frameworks could be enormous and daunting (Loe 2004). The assumption that sexual beliefs and experiences of young and old should always be in accordance with obtainable norms and values within time and space have been challenged with findings from existing research. Such expectations are cultural stereotypes and ideologies constructed and reconstructed through historical processes (Ikpe 2004). Ironically, presumptions like this are translated into the various forms of care and support available to meet the sexual health needs of the old

(Gott and Hinchliff 2003; Watters and Boyd 2009). Within biomedicine, aging is depicted as a risky and vulnerable process that demands constant surveillance (Katz and Marshall 2003). The promise of life extension within a bio-gerontological framework has been criticized for its emphasis on biology and technology without recognizing the interpretative understanding of aging and old age (Vincent 2006; Vincent *et al.* 2008). From a structuration perspective, social actors possess the capacity to influence the social structures through various forms of interaction and vice versa (Giddens 1984). The aged are active social actors within their cultures (Fox 2005), but sexuality issues in the sociology of aging are left on the peripheral (Arber *et al.* 2007). Thus, the practices and experiences related to sexuality in later life are worth discussing as each stage of sexual development has its own tasks and outcomes (Levy 1994; Sharpe 2003; Weeks 2003).

Studies on sexuality in old age suggest that elderly persons appreciate their sexual health and want to keep on enjoying their sexuality (Gott and Hinchliff 2003; Nusbaum and Hamilton 2002). However, the sexualization of the aging process has implications in later life for both the individual and the society. Exploring the presumed consensus or the struggle with normative values will require an understanding of the sexual beliefs and experiences of the adults themselves. Beliefs and practices are inseparable from the large social and epistemological orders from which they derive their significance (Katz 1996: 39). Ageism, which is a negative attitude towards older people or the elderly, has the potential to erode the psychosocial benefits which might accrue to older adults enjoying their sexual health to an advanced age. Older adults may be self-conscious about how they express their sexuality. Contradictions at this level could create regrets, shame, depression, and disappointments with one's self (Agunbiade *et al.* 2011).

Cultural beliefs, masculinity and medicine use

Cultural beliefs are the ideals and thoughts that influence the thinking and social interactions of individual members of a group with others (among themselves, their gods and other groups). In addition, cultural beliefs could serve as guiding principles for interested subscribers to adopt as signposts (Plog 1980). From the rationalist perspective, compliance or non-compliance with normative expectations is part of the observable properties of social existence (Clayton 2010; Otite and Ogionwo 2006). Such expectations are however, gendered and unequal. Among the Yoruba people, there are proverbs portraying exemplary lifestyles within and across gender as hallmarks of good old age (Owomoyela 2005). For instance, within the social field of sexual desires and expressions, the male gender is advantaged. Right from infanthood to adulthood, boys and girls are differently socialized, which shapes both their day-to-day lives and marital relations (Fadipe 1970). Within this social framework, the males are socially allowed to explore their sexual desires and pleasures and probably sample as many women as possible. While this may not be stated in explicit terms, gender biases are often brought to bear when a woman protests against her husband's or fiancé's infidelity or extramarital relations.

Despite the influence of culture, globalization has contributed to the changing face of what may be described as African sexualities (Tamale 2011). In recent times, foreign pharmaceutical remedies for sexual enhancement have become popular alongside the traditional herbal medicine. Prior to the importation of western medicine to the African society, traditional medicine existed as an institution and profession charged with the provision of health care (Konadu 2007; Oyebola 1980). African traditional medicine differs philosophically and in practice from western medicine (Keller 1978). Medicine is central among Africans. It represents anything that has the ability to effect a change anyhow, anywhere and anytime (Keller 1978). African traditional medicine has diverse remedies for different conditions, including conditions that may defy empirical investigation using the methodology of biomedicine (Jegede 2010; Oloyede 2010). A more pronounced aspect of the African traditional medicine is the use of herbal remedies. There are herbal remedies that aim at enhancing sexual performance throughout the life course as well as slowing down the aging process. Some of these remedies are for reproduction and pleasure purposes (Jegede 2010). To date, traditional medicine has remained relevant in meeting both health and psychosocial needs of the African people (Jegede 2010).

With cultural support for sexual enhancement and modification of the aging process already existing, the consumption of modern medicine for similar purposes came with ease. Complementing this is the culture of self-medication, which is prevalent in many Nigerian communities (Brieger *et al.* 2004). With unrestricted sale of sexuopharmaceuticals to both old and young, it is surprising that the experiences of middle-aged and older males using these drugs have been neglected by researchers. An interrogation of the experiences associated with sexuopharmaceutical drugs within a cultural context has implications for healthy aging. The realities of masculinity, sexuality and aging experiences are driven by cultural beliefs, values and practices (Gott and Hinchliff 2004; Rubinstein 1990; Weeks 2003). Hence, this study explores the beliefs and experiences of middle-aged and older Yoruba men within polygynous relations.

The study

Methodology

The study was conducted in Ibadan, one of the largest cities in Nigeria and the West African region. The city is largely an indigenous urban one, with representation of virtually all the major Nigerian ethnic groups. The research design was exploratory and based on qualitative approach. Qualitative methods are useful techniques for generating in-depth insights into realities, especially those that are difficult to quantify (Bowling 2002; Silverman 2000).

A snowball sampling strategy was adopted in recruiting men in polygynous marriages, while purposive sampling was employed in the recruitment of the doctors and nurses. The snowball sampling technique is useful in accessing populations that are somewhat hidden or difficult for researchers to access (Marshall and Rossman 1995). The recruitment of participants was restricted to Adeoyo-Mapo area of Ibadan, a core traditional area with high dominance of Yoruba indigenes. As shown from a study on determinants of households' residential districts' preferences within Metropolitan City of Ibadan, more indigenes of Ibadan reside in Adeoyo- Mapo area (Sanni and Akinyemi 2009). The area has a number of public and private hospitals among which is the Oyo State Hospital, a secondary tier hospital.

Entry into the community was facilitated through *gatekeepers*. In qualitative research, 'gatekeepers' could be individuals or departments who have control over subjects of interest. They often serve as an avenue to securing access to your subjects, thereby paving the way for good rapport (Devers and Frankel 2000). Four *gatekeepers* familiar with men in polygynous marriages were recruited within the community to identify the initial participants. Thereafter, the initial participants assisted by identifying friends with similar characteristics. This went on until twenty-six such participants were recruited. Five hospitals (two public and three private) were frequently mentioned by the participants. From these hospitals, nurses and doctors who had interacted with at least one married Yoruba man (50–75 years) within the previous six months were approached for voluntary participation.

With the assistance of the four gatekeepers and after briefing on the research objectives, face-to-face in-depth interviews were held with twenty-six Yoruba men (50–75 years) in polygynous marriages. Twelve interviews were held with eight nurses and four medical doctors who had relevant contact with middle-aged or older aged patients and had worked at the general outpatient units for five years or more. The interviews with the twenty-six Yoruba men were focused on their views on masculinity, sexuality, aging and their experiences with the use of modern medicine. The interview questions included: what does it mean to be a man in Yoruba culture? What are the differences in being married to one woman compared to marrying more than one woman? How should a wife respond to frequent sexual requests from her husband? In terms of sexual relations, what do you expect from your wives? In terms of sexual relations what do you think your wives expect from you as their husband? Additional interviews were also conducted among doctors and nurses with a focus on their views on medicine use and sexuality in old age.

Prior to the study, the interview guide was pre-tested among four Yoruba men (50–75 years) who were not included in this study. Three experienced male fieldworkers with an average age of 54 years were trained with the research instrument. The average length of the interviews ranged from 52 minutes to one hour 20 minutes. The interviews were conducted in locations preferred by the participants and considered conducive for them. This provided a convenient environment for interactive discussions. The interviews were conducted in the Yoruba language as preferred by some of the participants. Findings from the pre-test assisted in restructuring ambiguous questions for clarity in the main study. In the main study, all the participants were briefed on the study objectives, consent sought and received before the commencement of any interview. Participants were fully informed of their rights to discontinue with the interview at any point (Strydom 2002). All the interviews were audio-taped with the consent of the participants. Before each discussion, written informed consent was obtained where possible, while verbal consent was obtained from participants who could not read or write due to literacy or sight problems. Participants were informed of their right to decline participation at any point in the discussions.

Data analysis

Based on Ryan and Bernard's (2003) suggestions, a thematic approach was adopted in the data analysis. Within this purview, the rationale was to make sense of the rich data in order to construct a sense of common themes, patterns and shared experiences (Marshall and Rossman 1995). Since the interviews with polygynous males were conducted in the Yoruba language, an initial transcription of the interviews was done in Yoruba and later translated to English. Both the Yoruba and English transcriptions and translations were later given to an expert in both languages to ensure proper and accurate translation. As the analysis progressed, each transcript was read; key quotes and explanations were noted and extracted from subsequent transcripts.

Socio-demographic profile of interviewees

An appreciable proportion (21) of the men in polygynous marriages had between two and four wives. Interviewees between 60 and 69 years of age had the highest number of wives and children. A summary of other socio-demographics of the two categories of interviewees is contained in Tables 8.1 and 8.2.

Findings

Five interconnected themes emerged: essentiality of maleness and manhood; the exemplary adult and sexually aging well; the connection between a healthy body and cautious enjoyment of sexuality; medicine use and addiction fears; and the effect of low-back chronic pain and arthritis. A narrative approach was adopted in presenting each theme while individual extracts were provided where necessary.

Table 8.1 Socio-demographic characteristics of polygynous men interviewed

Variable	Participants' age (years)			Total (N=26)
	50–59	60–69	70+	
No. of wives				
2–4	9(43%)	8(38%)	4(19%)	21
5+	–	4(80%)	1(20%)	5
No. of living children				
5–10	4(50%)	3(38%)	1(12%)	8
11+	5(28%)	9(50%)	4(22%)	18
Religion				
Christianity	3(33%)	4(44%)	2(22%)	9
Islam	6(35%)	9(53%)	2(12%)	17
Educational status				
Minimum education*	8(50%)	5(31%)	3(19%)	16
Without education**	–	2(40%)	3(60%)	5

* Participants who had at least primary education and can read or write in Yoruba or English.
** Participants without primary education and can neither read nor write in Yoruba or English.

Essentiality of maleness and manhood

The participants described masculinity as essential in every domain of a man's life, particularly his sexuality and quality of marital relations. The dominant markers of masculinity include living to an advanced age, having sexual desires according to cultural standards, positive social outlooks and the absence of sexually transmitted infections. In heterosexual relations, the performance of masculinity – equated to maleness or manhood – requires active engagement in health and related practices that would ensure the constant sexual satisfaction of both the man and the woman. Good health, described as the absence of disease given support from medical systems, was identified as central in achieving this social image. Both the men in polygynous marriages and the healthcare professionals expressed the view that penetrative sex is a culturally acceptable way of demonstrating maleness or manhood. One of the doctors interviewed emphasized that it shows 'you are in-charge during sexual intercourse'. The description of sexuality expressed by the interviewees, with its focus on penile penetration and heterosexuality, may be described as hegemonic masculinity that leaves little consideration for the desires and satisfaction of the female gender.

Twenty of the participants shared the view that women appreciate penile penetration as a means of attaining sexual satisfaction in heterosexual relations. The participants argued that 'to satisfy a woman, a man must be strong and last during intercourse'. This position may be based on the

Table 8.2 Socio-demographic characteristics of doctors and nurses interviewed

Variable	Doctors	Nurses	Total (N=12)
Sex			
Male	4(33%)	8(67%)	12
Age (years)			
40–45	1(25%)	3(75%)	4
46–52	3(38%)	5(62%)	8
Religion			
Christianity	3(38%)	5(62%)	8
Islam	1(25%)	3(75%)	4
Educational status			
Below first degree*	–	6(100%)	6
Above first degree**	4(67%)	2(33%)	6
Marital status			
Married	3(25%)	9(75%)	12
Divorcee	1(100%)	–	1
Type of marriage			
Monogamy	4(36%)	7(64%)	11
Polygyny	–	1(100%)	1

* Below first degree (4 years in university).
** Above first degree (more than 4 years in university).

assumption that men have good understanding of their wives sexuality, but the reality is that this might not be a true reflection of the women's desire. Women's sexuality differs significantly from that of men (Schatzel-Murphy et al. 2009). Studies have shown that a number of Nigerian men believe they can think for their wives as well as themselves. Often, this creates strains and tensions in marriages (Bove and Valeggia 2009). An explanation for this might be found in the socialization process influencing who a man or woman should be. Through the socialization process, men are inculcated with the idea that satisfaction in sexual relations is based on penile penetration and strong erections. In the Yoruba cultural worldview, a man who wants to enjoy his sexual acts needs to take foods, herbs or any culturally approved substance to enhance their physical and mental strength (Agunbiade et al. 2011).

A less vocal but salient position was the fear that some women would engage in extramarital affairs if their husbands failed to satisfy them sexually. Five men related stories of this nature, where women had affairs because their own husbands were 'weak sexually'. While this may not be representative of all cases, the men argued that marital infidelity is multi-causal, but sexual satisfaction and economic consideration are critical.

> I know of a woman whose husband's personal driver has been having sexual affairs with [her] for more than four years now.
> (Polygynous male, aged 61)

> When I was much younger a number of my girl friends respect[ed] me and kept coming even after they had married because I know how to do it (penile intercourse) very well.
> (Polygynous male, aged 52)

The exemplary adult and sexually aging well

The health caregivers shared a stereotyped construct of exemplary adults in relation to sexuality in later life. To some of the health professionals, older males would be viewed as having sexually 'aged well' when they are able to minimize their desires and interest in sexual intercourse. When such desires and satisfaction are inevitable, it is gender biased and only permissive within heterosexual relations.

> Culturally, older adults that are 70 years and above, especially the women are to pay more attention to meeting their social responsibilities as 'grandpa' and 'grandma'. Nevertheless, so many 'grandpas' today are still very active. I am aware of two whose young wives gave birth two months ago.
> (Doctor, aged 43)

Similarly, one of the nurses interviewed argued that:

> The little energy shared on sexual activities in old age should rather be devoted to meaningful events such as community service or religious activities.
> (Nurse, aged 48)

While the need to increase relevance in old age by participating in community and religious activities was not refuted by the polygynous men, they felt that involvement in these activities should not deny them the pleasure of post-reproductive sexual activities. An interviewee eulogized the relevance of community participation through a Yoruba proverb:

> *A k í dúró nílùú ká fara hẹ.* One must live as a part of one's community.[1]
> (Polygynous male, aged 68)

A common position among the polygnous men was that only frail men who have lost their strength due to poverty, failing health and reckless lifestyle would not be able to perform sexually again at the age of 60–70 years.

I can't remember the last time I struggled to feel moved towards my wives. I have good ways of taking care of myself. I hardly eat sugary things that could reduce my sexual strength even at this age. I have both western and traditional doctors as friends and I use both medicines in keeping myself fit.

(Polygynous male, aged 69)

A number of young males have lost their manhood – that is ability to satisfy a woman sexually due to reckless lifestyle.

(Polygynous male, aged 72)

With a healthy body, there is no harm but enjoyment with caution

While a number of the polygynous men acknowledged their continuous desires for sexual activities, the participants debunked *ad infinitum* indulgence. This was hinged on the fact that life itself is finite and may require some level of dynamism especially with aging bodies, failing health and dwindling informal social support. They agreed that sexual activities in later life could decline drastically, especially with ailing health and other life challenges. On this basis, the Yoruba philosophy of *jeje laiye gba* (humility and patience are the virtues for good living) was reiterated among the older (70 years and above) polygynous men. To this category of interviewees, an individual being bestowed with good health in old age transcends the issue of lifestyle alone. It depends on multiple factors including one's *ori* (inner head) and other external factors.

Àlàáfíà baba eṣo; ojúrírí baba ara líle. Well-being, father of commanding presence; peace of mind, father of well-being.

(Polygynous male, aged 74)

Medicine use and addiction fears

The availability of traditional Yoruba medicine aimed towards modifying the aging process as well as improving penetrative sex may have supported the increasing patronage of modern medicine for similar purposes as well as improving penetrative sex. A number of the polygynous men argued that, as one ages, declining performance measured in terms of penetrative heterosexual relations is increasingly common. As a coping measure, self-medication and plural medicine use were common practices. Various information sources on how to improve health and sexual performance were referred to. Prominent among these sources were peers, patent medicine vendors, neighbours, and traditional and modern medical practitioners.

With the practice of plural medication, the interviewees compared the access and affordability of western medication to traditional Yoruba medicine. While therapies from both medical systems differ in orientation and applications, the polygynous men believed both are complementary but decisions on which to use are contingent on the perceived problem at hand. With the wide use and acceptance of medicine in old age, the interviewees complained of fake drugs and the difficulties in accessing prescribed medications when needed, especially at patent medicine shops.

Patent medicine vendors are widely available and enjoy high patronage in many Nigerian communities (Brieger et al. 2004). Despite the challenges, the participants admitted that sexuopharmaceutical drugs are relatively available in some patent shops. However, the men complained of fear of stigma as they prefer the use of terminologies such as 'action drugs' when asking vendors for such drugs. This experience was not peculiar to the older men; there were occasions when some of the middle-aged men would prefer to send a young person around to the medicine vendor shops using a description instead of the real brand of the drug.

The interviewees expressed concern over the plausibility of addiction as well as the side effects that may manifest in the distant future. The fear of side effects occurred more in the interviews with the healthcare professionals. This was related to the self-medication practices common with many adults in the community. The doctors warned against an impending problem in this area as many older people in particular lack support for their health needs. The healthcare practitioners observed that a number of older males delay coming for medical attention except when forced by ailing health or by their significant others.

Low-back chronic pain and arthritis

Having acknowledged the relevance of good health as essential to sexual activities in old age, some of the polygynous men complained about occasional low-back chronic pain and arthritis. In addition, they expanded on how this affects their quality of life and sexuality. Among the middle-aged men, some of these problems were attributed to biological and occupational hazards in particular and not to their indulgence in sexual activities. However, a slight shift was observed in the experiences of older men. Among this latter category, persistent low-back chronic pain and arthritis were occasionally interpreted as signs of old age that have affected their sexual health and quality of marital relations to varying extents. Plural medications, especially through peer referrals and self-administration, were common sources of help among the men. Visiting a modern healthcare practitioner was infrequently compared to self-medication. A number of the men (middle-aged and older) lamented the wasting of time and the lack of adequate attention to their health needs at the available public hospitals. The few who patronize both private and public hospitals believed more attention and privacy are available in private hospitals. On a few occasions, especially when they were ill, some of the doctors in private hospitals have inquired about their sexual health.

Discussion of findings

This chapter presents the cultural constructions of masculinity, aging, sexuality and the experiences associated with the use of modern medicine among polygynous Yoruba men alongside the views of modern health caregivers. Face-to-face in-depth interviews provided insights into the worldview of the men (50–75 years) and that of the health caregivers. Masculinity was portrayed as essential to success in every sphere of life including intimate relations. As described by Salamone (2010: 145), within the Yoruba worldview, men are differentiated from boys based on acts and practices. A man can be likened to a woman based on acts and practices that have been described as feminine. In everyday practices, men are expected to depict or exert their masculinity in their interactions with their fellow men and women. Throughout the participants' narratives, the ability to demonstrate masculinity at all times brings personal and social satisfaction. This supports the multi-dimensionality of masculinity and suggests how social actors struggle to connect with cultural ideals of maleness within time and space (Connell 1995; Calasanti and King 2005).

The emphasis on acts and practices that are domineering reflects the unequal power relations in polygynous marriage. This may also indicate lack of effective communication even in intimate acts like intercourse. The age gap between most husbands and their wives in polygyous marriages, supported by the cultural position that women should be submissive, may have been a further boost to the men's ego as they negotiated their wives' sexual satisfaction. While a number of the men may be having their way with their wives, it is likely that their wives would want to conform just to achieve other things from their husbands. Bove and Valeggia (2009) have described polgynous marriage in African society as 'co-operative conflicts within households'.

With the proposition among the participants that marital infidelity may be associated with sexual dissatisfaction with one's partner, a number of the men were eager to protect and boost penile penetration with the use of medicine as they aged with a number of younger wives. This finding adds to the existing research on the factors associated with extramarital affairs among Nigerian men (Oyediran et al. 2010). Sexual dissatisfaction with one's partner was not asked about in the Demographic Health Survey data that was used by Oyediran et al. (2010); but the fear of losing a wife(s) to an energetic man who may possess more sexual prowess may have an effect on the participants themselves as there might be pressure to consume sexuopharmaceutical drugs. The temptation to over-consume anti-aging medicine and the effects on healthy aging could be described as one of the inherent contradictions with anti-aging medicine (Katz and Marshall 2003; Mykytyn 2008). Faced with the physiological state of aging bodies, the fear of disappointing a woman through 'low sexual performance' and the promises of anti-aging medicine, use of the latter may be enticing.

In view of the above, contradictory positions emerged between the polygynous men and the health caregivers. From a professional perspective, the healthcare givers portrayed aging as a critical period that calls for caution and surveillance. This position was substantiated with a cultural ideal of exemplary adults, as the healthcare providers admonished older men to focus on essential social responsibilities rather than utilizing their energy on sexual activities. This contradicts the views of the polygynous men, who interpreted the need to constantly satisfy their wives sexually as a mission that calls for support from medical systems. Some studies have argued that age, similar to gender, establishes a particular order (Twigg 2004) and it is one of the reasons for discriminatory and oppressive practices (Calasanti 2007; Calasanti and Slevin 2006). The contradictions between the views of health professionals and lay people on sexual health- related behaviour has implications for the therapeutic encounters and the quality of care available to this category of adults (Gott and Hinchliff 2003), especially in the prevention of sexually transmitted infections. The position that the sexual needs of adults may not be essential to achieving a healthy aging population is limiting since older adults themselves perceive their sexual needs as an essential dimension of health in later life (Watters and Boyd 2009).

In contrast to the healthcare givers' fear, the polygynous men decried the difficulties in accessing some essential medications. Inadequate availability of essential drugs is common with the delivery of modern healthcare services in Nigeria and in the sub-Saharan Africa in general (African Regional Health Report 2006). This may be contributing to the continuous preference for self-medication and patronage of plural medical systems in Nigeria (Brieger *et al.* 2004; Jegede 2002). Similar to the problem of non-availability of prescribed drugs is the problem of importation of fake drugs. While the National Agency for Food and Drug Administration and Control (*NAFDAC*) has been very forceful in addressing the problem of fake drugs, the continuous reliance on importation of drugs and the inadequate monitoring of patent medicine sellers will continue to create challenges in meeting the health needs of the Nigerian populace.

Both the polygynous men and the healthcare givers were wary of the risk of addiction with sexuopharmaceutical drugs. This was expected from the polygynous men as they are experienced users and must have noticed some changes in their sexual activities and body as a whole. This may be added to findings from western studies on the pleasures and perceived dangers in the use of Viagra, one of the most widely publicized sexuopharmaceutical drugs (Loe 2004; Potts *et al.* 2003).

The description of sexuality within the framework of penile penetration and heterosexuality by the polygynous men and the healthcare providers may be described as hegemonic masculinity. This leaves little considerations for the desires and satisfaction of the female gender, even though the females are critical stakeholders in heterosexual relations. Potts *et al.* (2003) have earlier established this situation, where a number of the women interviewed shared their disappointments and mixed feelings about the centrality of Viagra and the marginalization of their desires and pleasures in their relationships with their spouse. While heterosexuality was dominant in the sexuality discourse and expectations of the participants, this does not negate the plausible existence of individuals or groups who may have sexual desires towards same sex or who are bisexual without disclosure of such identity.

Findings from this study are limited as the focus was on a relatively small sample of polygynous men in heterosexual relationships. Capturing the views and experiences of wives of the polygynous men could have provided additional insights, but this is a topic for another study. Despite the limitations, this study is the first to examine the intersection of masculinity, aging, medicine use and sexuality among middle-aged and older Yoruba men.

In conclusion, the availability of anti-aging medicine provides additional opportunities and challenges for the men in polygynous marriage to redefine their mind and bodily experiences in line with cultural notions of masculinity. Given the popularity of patent medicine vendors, the increasing circulation of sexuopharmaceutical drugs and suggestions of potential abuse by adolescent and young people in some studies (Bowleg et al. 2011; Groes-Green 2009), there are numerous questions raised about health implications. Going by the experiences of the polygynous men, especially in relation to their use of medicine in sexual practices, there are chances of latent health challenges that may be associated with their use of sexual enhancement drugs with or without prescriptions. The situation could be worsened by the low health literacy rate among older adults in Nigeria. With the proliferation of substandard drugs in Nigeria, despite the efforts of the NAFDAC, addressing health literacy among Nigerian populace would make consumers more informed to engage in healthy practices that will be beneficial to their health and the society.

The availability of age-friendly primary care systems, as prescribed by the World Health Organization (2004), and the willingness of health caregivers to engage old and older adults in constructive sexual discourse without prejudice would be relevant in promoting sexual health in later life. In addition, commitment to rights-based provision of sexual health services would further assist in meeting and promoting the sexual health needs of the aged.

Notes

1 All the proverbs were provided by the interviewees, while the widely accepted forms and interpretations were from Owomoyela (2005) as cited in the reference.

References

Adebusoye, L. A., Ladipo, M. M., Owoaje, E. T., and Ogunbode, A. M. (2011) 'Morbidity pattern amongst elderly patients presenting at a primary care clinic in

Nigeria', *African Journal of Primary Health and Family Medicine*: http://www.ajol.info/index.php/nmp/article/viewFile/28945/38085 (accessed Aug. 2011).

African Regional Health Report (2006) http://whqlibdoc.who.int/afro/2006/9290231033_rev_eng.pdf (accessed Sept. 2007).

Agunbiade, O. M., Titilayo, A., and Opatola, M. (2011) 'Cultural beliefs and concerns for healthy sexuality in late life among Yoruba adults in South West Nigeria', in B. Worsfold (ed.), *Acculturating Age: Approaches to Cultural Gerontology* (pp. 33–59), Lleida, Spain: University of Lleida.

Alex, L., Hammarstrom, A., Norberg, A., and Lundman, B. (2008) 'Construction of masculinities among men aged 85 and older in the north of Sweden', *Journal of Clinical Nursing*, 17(4): 451–9.

Arber, S., Andersson, L., and Hoff, A. (2007) 'Changing approaches to gender and ageing: Introduction', *Current Sociology*, 55(2): 147–53.

Asuquo, A. (1999) 'Extramarital sexual behaviour in a Nigerian urban centre', *Journal of Marriage and Family*, 21(3): 110–21.

Bauer, M., McAuliffe, L., and Rhonda, N. (2007) 'Sexuality, health care and the older person: An overview of the literature', *International Journal of Older People Nursing*, 2(1): 63–8.

Bekibele, C. O., and Gureje, O. (2010) 'Fall incidence in a population of elderly persons in Nigeria', *Gerontology*, 56(3): 278–83.

Bennett, K. M. (2007) '"No sissy stuff": Towards a theory of masculinity and emotional expression in older widowed men', *Journal of Aging Studies*, 21: 347–56.

Bove, R., and Valeggia, C. (2009) 'Polygyny and women's health in sub-Saharan Africa', *Social Science and Medicine*, 68: 21–9.

Bowleg, L., Teti, M., Massie, J. S., Patel, A., Malebranche, D. J., and Tschann, J. M. (2011) '"What does it take to be a man? What is a real man?" Ideologies of masculinity and HIV sexual risk among Black heterosexual men', *Culture, Health and Sexuality*, 13(5): 545–59.

Bowling, A. (2002) *Research Methods in Health: Investigating Health and Health Services*, Buckingham: Open University Press.

Brieger, W. R., Osamor, P. E., Salami, K. K., Oladepo, O., and Otusanya, S. A. (2004) 'Interactions between patent medicine vendors and customers in urban and rural Nigeria', *Health Policy and Planning*, 19(3): 177–82.

Butler, J. (1990) *Gender Trouble: Feminism and the Subversion of Identity*, New York: Routledge.

Calasanti, T. M. (2004) 'Feminist gerontology and old men', *Journal of Gerontology: Social Sciences*, 6: 305–14.

Calasanti, T. M. (2007) 'Bodacious berry, potency wood and the aging monster: Gender and age relations in anti-aging ads', *Social Forces*, 86(1): 335–55.

Calasanti, T., and King, N. (2005) 'Firming the floppy penis: Age, class, and gender relations in the lives of old men', *Men and Masculinities*, 8(1): 3–23.

Calasanti, T., and Slevin, K. (eds) (2006) *Age Matters: Realigning Feminist Thinking*, London: Routledge.

Clayton, B. (2010) 'Re-evaluating difference in light of biology's intriguing linguistic compliance', *Current Sociology*, 58(6): 859–78.

Connell, R. W. (1995) *Masculinities*, Los Angeles, CA: Polity Press.

Devers, K. J., and Frankel, R. M. (2000) 'Study design in qualitative research 2: Sampling and data collection strategies', *Education for Health*, 13(2): 263–71.

Fadipe, N. A. (1970) *The Sociology of the Yoruba*, Ibadan: Ibadan University Press.
Falen, D. J. (2008) 'Polygyny and Christian marriage in Africa: the case of Benin'. *African Studies Review*, 51(2): 51-74.
Foucault, M. (1990) *The History of Sexuality: The Use of Pleasure*, New York: Vantage Books.
Fox, N. J. (2005) 'Cultures of ageing in Thailand and Australia. (What can an ageing body do?)', *Sociology*, 39(3): 481–98.
Giddens, A. (1984) *The Constitution of Society*, Cambridge: Polity Press.
Gott, M., and Hinchliff, S. (2003) 'How important is sex in later life? The views of older people', *Social Science and Medicine*, 56: 1617–28.
Groes-Green, C. (2009) 'Hegemonic and subordinated masculinities: Class, violence and sexual performance among young Mozambican men', *Nordic Journal of African Studies*, 18(4): 286–304.
Hollos, M., Larsen, U., Obono, O., and Whitehouse, B. (2009) 'The problem of infertility in high fertility populations: Meanings, consequences and coping mechanisms in two Nigerian communities', *Social Science and Medicine*, 68: 2061–8.
Igenoza, A. O. (2007) *Polygamy and the African Churches: A Biblical Appraisal of an African Marriage System*, Ibadan: African Association for the Study of Religion, the Nigerian Publication Bureau.
Ikpe, E. B. (2004). *Human Sexuality in Nigeria: A Historical Perspective*, African Regional Sexuality Resource Centre: http://www.arsrc.org/downloads/uhsss/ikpe.pdf (accessed Dec. 2006).
Izugbara, C. O. (2001) 'Tasting the forbidden fruits: The social context of debut sexual encounters among young persons in a rural Nigerian community', *The African Anthropologist*, 8(1): 96–107.
Jegede, A. S. (2002) 'The Yoruba cultural construction of health and illness', *Nordic Journal of African Studies*, 11(3): 322–35.
Jegede, O. (2010) *Incantations and Herbal Cures in Ifa Divination: Emerging Issues in Indigenous Knowledge*, Ibadan: African Association for the Study of Religion, the Nigerian Publication Bureau.
Kampf, A., and Botelho, L. A. (2009) 'Anti-aging and biomedicine: Critical studies on the pursuit of maintaining, revitalizing and enhancing aging bodies', *Medicine Studies*, 1: 187–95.
Katz, S. (1996) *Disciplining Old Age: The Formation of Gerontological Knowledge*, London: University Press of Virginia.
Katz, S., and Marshall, B. (2003) 'New sex for old: Lifestyle, consumerism, and the ethics of aging well', *Journal of Aging Studies*, 17: 3–16.
Keller, B. B. (1978) 'Marriage and medicine: Women's search for love and luck', *African Social Research*, 24: 489–505.
Konadu, K. (2007) *Indigenous Medicine and Knowledge in African Society*, New York: Routledge.
Levy, J. A. (1994). 'Sex and sexuality in later life stages', in A. S. Rossi (ed.), *Sexuality across the Life Course* (pp. 287–309), Chicago, IL: University of Chicago Press.
Loe, M. (2004) 'Sex and the senior woman: Pleasure and danger in the Viagra era', *Sexualities*, 7(3): 303–26.
Marshall, C., and Rossman, G. B. (1995) *Designing Qualitative Research*, 2nd edn, Thousand Oaks, CA: Sage.
Mykytyn, C. E. (2008) 'Medicalizing the optimal: Anti-aging medicine and the quandary of intervention', *Journal of Aging Studies*, 22(4): 313–21.

Nusbaum, M. R. H., and Hamilton, C. D. (2002) 'The proactive sexual health history', *American Family Physician*, 66(9): 1705–12.
Olawoye, J. E., Omololu, F. O., Aderinto, Y., Adeyefa, I., Adeyemo, D., and Osotimehin, B. (2004) 'Social construction of manhood in Nigeria: Implications for male responsibility in reproductive health', *African Population Studies*, 19(2): 1–20.
Oloyede, O. (2010) 'Epistemological issues in the making of an African medicine: Sutherlandia (Lessertia Frutescens)', *African Sociological Review*, 14(2): 74–88.
Otite, O., and Ogionwo, W. (2006) *An Introduction to Sociological Studies*, 2nd edn, Ibadan: Heinemann Educational Books.
Owomoyela, O. (2005) *Yoruba Proverbs*, Lincoln, NE: University of Nebraska Press.
Oyebola, D. D. O. (1980) '*Traditional medicine* and its practitioners *among* the Yoruba of Nigeria: A classification', *Social Science and Medicine*, 14A: 23–9.
Oyediran, K., Isiugo-Abanihe, U. C., Feyisetan, B.J. and Ishola, G. P. (2010) 'Prevalence of and factors associated with extramarital sex among Nigerian men', *American Journal of Mens Health*, 4: 124–134.
Plog, F. (1980) *Anthropology: Decisions, Adaptation, and Evolution*, New York: Alfred A. Knopf.
Potts, A., Gavey, N., Grace, V. M., and Vares, T. (2003) 'The downside of Viagra: Women's experiences and concerns', *Sociology of Health and Illness*, 25(7): 697–719.
Rosaldo, M. Z., and Lamphere, L. (1974) *Woman, Culture and Society*, Stanford, CA: Stanford University Press.
Rubinstein, R. L. (1990) 'Nature, culture, gender, age: A critical review', in R. L. Rubinstein (ed.), *Anthropology and Aging* (pp. 109–28), Dordrecht: Kluwer Academic Publishers.
Ryan, G. W., and Bernard, H. R. (2003) 'Techniques to identify themes', *Field Methods*, 15(1): 85–109.
Salamone, F. (2010) 'The depiction of masculinity in classic Nigerian literature', in H. Bloom (ed.), *Bloom's Modern Critical Interpretations: Chinua Achebe's Things Fall Apart* (pp. 141–52), New York: Infobase Publishing.
Sanni, L., and Akinyemi, F. O. (2009) 'Determinants of households' residential districts' preferences within Metropolitan City of Ibadan, Nigeria', *Journal of Human Ecology*, 25(2): 137–41.
Schatzel-Murphy, E. A., Harris, D. A., Knight, R. A., and Milburn, M. A. (2009) 'Sexual coercion in men and women: Similar behaviors, different predictors', *Archives of Sexual Behaviors*, 38: 974–86.
Sharpe, T. H. (2003) 'Adult sexuality', *Family Journal*, 11(4): 420–6.
Silverman, D. (2000) *Doing Qualitative Research: A Practical Handbook*, Thousand Oaks, CA: Sage.
Strydom, H. (2002) 'Ethical aspects of research in the social sciences and human services professions', in H. de Vos, A. S. Strydom, C. B. Fouche, and C. S. L. Delport (eds), *Research at Grassroots: A Primer for the Social Sciences and Human Service Professions* (pp. 62–76), Pretoria: Van Schaik Publishers.
Tamale, S. (2011) 'Researching and theorising sexualities in Africa', in S. Tamale (ed.), *African Sexualities: A Reader*, Cape Town: Pambazuka Press.
Thompson, E. H. (1994) 'Older men as invisible in contemporary society', in E. H. Thompson (ed.), *Older Men's Lives* (pp. 1–21), Thousand Oaks, CA: Sage.

Twigg, J. (2004) 'The body, gender, and age: Feminist insights in social gerontology', *Journal of Aging Studies*, 18(1): 59–73.
Vincent, J. A. (2006) 'Ageing contested: Anti-ageing science and the cultural construction of old age', *Sociology*, 40(4): 681–98.
Vincent, J. A., Tulle, E., and Bond, J. (2008) 'The anti-ageing enterprise: Science, knowledge, expertise, rhetoric and values', *Journal of Aging Studies*, 22: 291–4.
Watters, Y., and Boyd, T. V. (2009) 'Sexuality in later life: Opportunity for reflections for healthcare providers', *Sexual and Relationship Therapy*, 24(3): 307–15.
Weeks, J. (2003) *Sexuality*, 2nd edn, London: Routledge.
West, C., and Zimmerman, D. H. (1987) 'Doing Gender', *Gender and Society*, 1: 125–51.
Willison, K., and Andrews, G. (2004) 'Complementary medicine and older people: Past research and future directions', *Complementary Therapies in Nursing and Midwifery*, 10: 80–91.
World Health Organisation (2004) *Active Ageing: Towards Age-Friendly Primary Health Care:* http://whqlibdoc.who.int/publications/2004/9241592184.pdf (accessed Nov. 2010).

9 'I haven't died yet'

Navigating masculinity, aging and andropause in Turkey

Maral Erol and Cenk Özbay

Men encounter varying crises regarding their masculinities throughout their life courses, such as the crossroads at when they cannot find a decent job and cannot maintain the 'breadwinner' position at home (McDowell 2003), or the watershed when they start college and endeavour to get in on fraternities and circles of friends (Kimmel 2009). Men would *normally* be expected to adapt their masculine identities to these changing conditions and when they fail to do so they are tagged as 'in crisis'. Men also face a crisis as they get older: andropause ('male climacteric' or 'the male menopause' or 'low testosterone') frames the current discourse of this moment of crisis that men at a certain age may experience.

In the broadest sense, masculinity is imagined and experienced through a set of tests, challenges, struggles and competitions that involve not only women, but also, more significantly, other men. Representations of masculinities across cultures depict this sense of exertion and strength. Hegemonic masculinity (Connell 1995) is symbolically constructed via these portrayals of frenetic power and boisterous success.[1] When the male subject fails to enact such hustle and bustle of virility, he is gradually deemed marginalized, dissident, excluded or subaltern; somehow lacking manhood, a wounded masculinity. Andropause poses this threat of losing masculinity; the sense of championship mislaid, through men's own bodies – somewhere the struggle is at its highest difficulty. Men encounter and strive to deal with the threat of losing their sense of masculine selves not from outside, but from inside, from the very source of their own manhood.[2]

This chapter examines how andropause is framed and analysed through the discourses of aging and masculinity in Turkey, where public debate about masculinity is yet to be matured and stabilized. First, we outline the discussions around andropause in the intersection of medicine, medical sociology and gender studies, and then we move on to locate specific uses of the term in popular discourses in Turkey.

Andropause: is it really 'male menopause'?

Early examples of the literature on medicalization and gender dynamics focus on women, and mostly consist of feminist critiques, with the argument that women's bodies (and particularly reproductive functions) are the principal site for medicalization and medical intervention. Examples include medicalization of childbirth and pregnancy (Rothman 1989), menstruation (Martin 1987), infertility (Inhorn 1994) and menopause (Guillemin 2000; Houck 2006; Lock 1993; Watkins 2007a). Social scientific narratives of medicalization of male bodies are more limited, and more recent, including the role of Viagra and its variants (Loe 2004; Wienke 2006; Marshall 2006), male aging and andropause (Marshall 2007, 2009; Conrad 2007; Szymczak and Conrad 2006), prostate cancer (Broom 2004; Oliffe 2005), disability (Gerschick and Miller 1994), and, more generally, relations between masculinity and health (Courtenay 2000; Sabo and Gordon 1995).

Andropause has a fluctuating, if not contested, medical history (see Watkins, this volume). Interest in male aging and therapies for rejuvenation was a popular subject in Western medicine in the late nineteenth century. However, male menopause disappeared from the medical radar as an aging issue till the end of twentieth century while the female climacteric was increasingly medicalized, until it reappeared in 1990s (Oudshoorn 1997; Szymczak and Conrad 2006; Watkins 2007b).

Within the social science literature on andropause, Conrad (2007) focuses on the role of pharmaceutical corporations in coming up with the medical category of andropause, while Marshall (2007) argues that medicalization of the aging male body is a result of cultural reconstruction rather than new scientific evidence. We agree with both of these statements, and would like to further this argument by showing how the cultural reconstruction of andropause can also include resistance to medicalization, by presenting the Turkish example.

In Turkey, the process of the medicalization of menopause triggered a similar vein of medicalizing discourse on the aging male body. Even though narratives of andropause suggest a biomedical approach to a (hormonal) change that men go through after middle age, it may not be correct to label this process as 'medicalization' of male aging per se.[3] Especially compared to the medicalization of menopause, this move toward popularization of andropause does not involve the necessity to be under medical supervision due to possible dangerous effects of 'the change', as was the case with women. While the leading emotion behind medicalization of menopause is fear (particularly of osteoporosis), the underlying emotions that accompany andropause are anxiety (over maintaining heterosexual virility, 'heteromasculinity') and shame (if the masculine subject fails to stay as virile as he was). There is also a considerable amount of tolerance for the predictable changes in behaviour that may come with the hormonal change, such as optimistically feeling more energetic and/or going after younger women.

Research on Turkish masculinities

Feminist thought and women's groups in Turkey were first to question men as gendered beings and the particular masculinities that men enacted as early as the late 1980s. A focus in the academy on men and masculinities within a gender studies framework came much later. The first significant compilation of research and meditation on men and masculinities in the Turkish language was published as a special issue of the leading social science journal *Toplum and Bilim* in 2004 (Sokmen 2004). Since then, researchers have written many books, journal articles, MA theses and PhD dissertations on masculinities in Turkey or about Turkish men in diaspora (see e.g. Aktas 2009; Atencio and Koca 2011; Basaran 2007; Bereket and Adam 2006; Bilgin 2004; Delice 2010; Ehrkamp 2008; Erol 2003; Ewing 2008; Kizilkan 2009; Özbay 2010a, 2010b; Sancar 2009; Sinclair-Webb 2006).[4]

This body of research and commentaries concentrated on a range of specific domains of Turkish masculinities. One of these areas that govern men's lives as gendered subjects is the relation between military institutions, regimes of state-sponsored modernity and the different instruments of the Turkish nation-state. The desire for and the disciplining processes of modernization and Westernization shaped and reshaped how men in Turkey saw themselves in a self-reflexive manner. Men were invited to play a constitutive role in the construction of the enlightened, decent citizen, 'the new Turkish man', by official state discourses and the multiple regulatory mechanisms including law and the army. The new Turkish man was responsible not only for transforming himself into a modern, Western, republican, secular, rational, educated, wilful subject but also for moulding people around him, such as his family, kin, friends and neighbours. When he could not perform as expected as the new man (or, when he resisted doing so), he was excluded from social and political relations and represented as the insular, dissident, backward – if not criminalized – subject, a sociopolitical pathology.

Another field of concentration in studies of men and masculinities in Turkey is the various sexual actions in which men engage. Documenting the discursive and spatial aspects of the counter-normative and dissident sexual subcultures (or queer sexualities) in Turkey was on the rise while, on the other hand, the detailed analysis of heterosexuality and its patterns of institutionalization were mostly absent. Although modern Turkish man was depicted as heterosexual, married with children, or moving along that path of reproduction in the official state discourses, the increasing power of global cosmopolitanism, tourism and tolerance for social diversity enabled sexual minorities to gain visibility and representation in the liberal discourses as one of the subaltern and disadvantaged group in society. However the complex interrelations among men, who embody diverse masculinities, are still relatively under-represented in public and academic discussions in relation to family issues and changing relations between women and men.

Men in Turkey are studied as a monolithic category without paying full attention to the inherent, intra-group distinctions that men can have. How different men are positioned in the social map of symbolic hierarchies based on their age, ethnicity, body, sexuality, class or location is mostly understudied. Instead, a well-rooted understanding that puts men and women – as two coherent, stable, mutually exclusive groups – in opposition and strives to elucidate gendered dynamics between the two sexes persists. Beyond this conventional view of the patriarchal sex-division, which is based on an unquestioned dichotomy between women and men, the ways in which certain domains of life, such as the economy, sports, popular culture and religion, affect and reconstruct men and masculinities in Turkey are also unexplored.

Hegemonic masculinity (Connell 1995) in Turkey is largely narrated through a holistic male sex identity that encompasses all males and not via specific masculine gendered practices, with the significant exception of effeminacy. In other words, all male bodies are automatically deemed to embody hegemonic Turkish masculinity without particular reference to how these men individually project their manhood in terms of bodily movements, gestures, social relations and subjectivity. In this context, hegemonic masculinity becomes an elusive concept, which sometimes overlaps with the classical patriarchal view (male domination over women), and fails to underline the differences and relations *between* men from a prism of power dynamics. Honour (*namus*) is highlighted as the cornerstone of Turkish masculinity and it is defined most commonly as the men's dominion over women's bodies. Given this insufficient focus on intricate power relations between men, we can conclude that hegemonic masculinity in Turkey is largely construed by means of representation of political figures, popular opinion leaders, celebrities and their lifestyles. The male body, its abilities and disabilities, certain illnesses (including AIDS) and the dynamics of aging (including andropause and erectile dysfunctions) are not among the concepts and issues that govern public and academic discussions on hegemonic masculinity in Turkey.

Masculinities and andropause

The *Oxford English Dictionary* defines andropause as 'a collection of symptoms, including fatigue and a decrease in libido, experienced by some older men and attributed to a gradual decline in testosterone levels', while it presents menopause as 'the period in a woman's life (typically between the ages of 45 and 50) when menstruation ceases'.[5] Even the simplest dictionary definitions of the two sexed terms for (more or less) the same life period do not match. Menopause is deemed as a threshold through which clear temporal distinctions apply: whether a biologically female body is in menopause or not. However, andropause is a more complicated case to investigate, identify and classify. It is indeed an *indeterminate* 'collection of symptoms' originated by the decrease of testosterone levels (if they decrease at all) that can be encountered by *some* men at different ages. In other words, andropause is a specific discourse that draws on ambiguous cultural and bodily narratives as they are reformulated and reproduced under the heavy influence of global pharmaceutical industry and the new privatized health regime.

The intersection between gender and health has long been analysed via women's bodies (Rosenfeld and Faircloth 2006). The relations between masculinity, health and the (male) body have primarily been explored through conceptions of risk, vulnerability and 'the costs of manhood' (Bourke 1996; Connell 1995, 2001; Messner 1997). Basically, there are diseases only men can have, such as prostate cancer, and diseases that men have a higher possibility of getting, for example, cardiovascular diseases. Masculine lifestyles in their hegemonic versions undermine job security and healthy diets and superimpose fast cars, heavy drinking, interpersonal violence, dangerous sports as well as embodied courageousness during war and military conflicts. Andropause, on the other hand, seems biogenic and thus independent from lifestyle choices that are regulated by hegemonic masculinity. It is seen as almost an arrival point that all men will eventually experience if they live long enough. Narratives of andropause are also contingent on men's fear of, and tendency to underestimate the pain and shame from, the physical symptoms they might experience. Men who enact, or endeavour to enact, hegemonic masculinity tend not to feel and talk about the processes that their bodies go through.

Maybe this reticence of men is the reason why the sociologist Don Sabo (2005: 336–40) in his review article did not include men in andropause in his list of 'male groups with special health needs'. He listed 'adolescent males, boys with ADHD, gay and bisexual men, infertile men, male athletes, male caregivers, male victims of sexual assault, men of color, and prisoners', without any reference either to 'aging men, old men' or 'men in andropause'. Despite the relative lack of academic interest in men in andropause within the field of masculinity studies, andropause is gaining visibility and recognition, especially through its link with erectile dysfunctions, the unstoppable rise of Viagra and other 'male enhancement drugs', the commodification of masculinity vis-à-vis surveillance, medical control and intervention. The male body in general has been progressively medicalized and andropause provides a significant niche in this trend with its concern with the two least contestable elements of masculinity: virility and potency.

In spite of the fact that men in andropause can be depicted with certain 'problems', such as drowsiness, lethargy, frailty, diffidence, atrophy and dilapidation at work, the most important single factor that characterizes andropause is sexuality. Lower libido and difficulty in having and sustaining erections mark the catastrophe of the almost-castrated man in andropause. In this sense, andropause matters because, more than anything else, it kills the potent man – the sexual male subject.

Discourses of andropause in Turkey

We have analysed a total of 247 articles and columns from five daily newspapers that are distributed nationally (namely *Akşam*, *Milliyet*, *Hürriyet*, *Sabah*, and *Zaman*) between the years 2000 and 2010. *Hürriyet* and *Sabah* are among the well-established and popular mainstream newspapers with high circulation figures. They cater to an imagined Turkish middle-class audience with a tendency to a central-right political viewpoint. Most of the articles in our sample came out of these two newspapers (95 articles from *Hürriyet* and 93 from *Sabah*). *Milliyet* is well known for its well-educated, urban, professional body of readers with central-left and secularist sensitivities. *Akşam* is a relatively young newspaper with lower circulation figures. *Zaman* is the most-read conservative, moderately Islamist newspaper, included for the sake of diversity in our sample.

Based on our analysis, there are roughly three main categories in the popular discourse on andropause in Turkey in the first decade of the twenty-first century. These categories are:

- andropause as a health problem;
- andropause as an explanation for marital infidelity or mid-life crisis;
- andropause as an insult.

The first of these categories relates to the medicalization of andropause by defining it as a medical problem, while the other two extrapolate on that 'medical' definition and combine it with the existing expectations and anxieties about masculinity. For all these categories, 2006 appears to be a turning point. Although andropause was mentioned in news stories (particularly health-related ones) before this date as well, there was an explosion in newspaper articles after this date, partly due to scandalous events that involved celebrities.[6] This led to discussions on what exactly andropause is, and whether or not it is different from more common conceptions of ordinary 'mid-life crisis'. Around the same time, a famous newspaper columnist, Selahattin Duman, introduced the derogatory term *azgın teke sendromu* (horny goat syndrome), in reference to male goats who start chasing young goats in the herd in their old age (Duman 2006). Although he stated that he does not believe in andropause, the term *azgın teke* came to be associated frequently with andropause, which contributed to the word andropause being used as an insult on its own. The popularity of andropause and *azgın teke* discussions in the media even led to a sarcastic pop song called 'Andropoz' (Andropause) in 2008, written and sung by Attila Atasoy, a middle-aged pop singer.

Framing andropause as a health problem

This category consists of news stories in the health/wellness sections of the newspapers, or interviews with the experts, mostly urologists or endocrinologists. The general narrative in these texts is that andropause is a health problem due to decreased levels of testosterone especially after the age of 40, although it does not necessarily happen to every man. Despite the fact that there are sub-categories within this group, like comparisons with menopause and mid-life crisis, the common point in all these stories is the medical language and reasoning evident in explanations.

The most typical example of this category is articles that try to answer the question 'What is andropause?' In these articles, andropause is defined as decrease in testosterone levels that can lead to symptoms like decreased libido, depression, weight gain, energy loss, decrease in muscle mass and sleep problems. In some stories, andropause is listed, yet not necessarily explained in detail, as one of the risks (or health problems) that come with aging.

There is usually stress on the symptoms of andropause as preventable, if a man takes care of himself properly and takes necessary precautions. The following is a quote from the mainstream newspaper *Hürriyet*, where Professor Akkus, a doctor interviewed regarding andropause, is answering the question 'What is this thing called andropause, or mid-life crisis?'

> Decrease in testosterone. Not just testosterone, but the change in the biologically active testosterone levels and the balance between testosterone and estrogen. With hypogonadism due to advanced age, testosterone decreases and the balance tips at the advantage of estrogen. This affects some men. It's not right to say 'Men have andropause'. Mid-life crisis is also a reflection of hormonal changes. Other psychological factors are probably effective as well. They have the anxiety of 'I'm running out of time. Am I missing the boat?' I should also emphasize that it's not correct to say 'His hormones have decreased, that's why he's in mid-life crisis.' Mid-life crisis occurs when the hormonal changes are added to the negative effects of economic and social state, decrease in work performance and some physical changes. Not all men necessarily go through andropause.
>
> (Ersan 2005)

So, andropause is certainly related to the change in hormone levels that comes with aging, however it does not negatively affect all men. It is important to note that the medical discourse presented here separates andropause (which is related to hormones) from mid-life crisis (which is a combination of hormone levels and outside factors). Medical doctors in particular endeavour to explain the possible differences between what is deemed as andropause and the symptoms of mid-life crisis.

The most frequently mentioned symptom of andropause is decreased libido, which is related to the mid-life crisis stories in the second category. Decreased libido is equated with the loss of masculine identity and most of the stories in this fashion stress the importance of sexual performance for a man's gender identity. Several stories cite the decrease in sexual desire and erotic performance as the reason for depression and irritability in andropause, and mention that this can lead to sexual adventures to prove one's manliness. Some articles, like the one below, cite the 'new woman' as a source of anxiety for an aging man, and offer medical assistance.

> When men want to be with a new woman, they get discouraged, especially if the woman is younger. Men coming from Anatolia feel the need to go through an andrological check-up and run to Prof. Dr. Halim Hattat to learn about their performance in bed generally when they are going to marry again and the new spouse is significantly younger. 'He is married, with several wives, and he is seventy years old. He wants to be with a new woman now. And we want to help him, because there is an interest, desire for sexuality here. If there is desire, we can help him, and increase his sexual performance regardless of his age.'
> (Kartal 1997)

This is an excerpt from an interview with Halim Hattat, who opened the Andrology Hospital (Hattat Özel Üro-Androloji Hastanesi) in Istanbul, and the aim of this interview is mostly to introduce the services provided by this new institution. It is also interesting that this interview was an earlier example of newspaper articles on andropause, taking place in 1997, before andropause became popular. Here we see a big emphasis on sexual desire in aging men, and a meticulously non-judgemental approach that prioritizes the demands of the applicants. However, there is also a disregard for the people he is interacting with, particularly the younger wives who are in an illegal (and unequal) polygynous relationship with the 70-year-old man in question.

An important sub-category of these stories is the comparison between menopause and andropause. Andropause is called 'male menopause' or 'male climacterium' in some of these stories, and in some others it is emphasized that andropause is different from female menopause. Another part of this comparison is the amount of attention that menopause receives in popular culture, and how andropause (and aging in men) is a relatively neglected topic. Osman Muftuoglu, a well-known doctor who has a standing column in the daily newspaper *Hürriyet*, touches upon this issue when commenting on the news stories written on andropause:

> Last week we lived through a serious 'andropause storm' that made quite a mess. Since the issue is related to sexuality and on top of that, is of concern to men, we shouldn't be surprised of the noise it made. Another reason of the storm is that Turkish society withheld the attention it freely gave to menopausal women from men. There are menopause societies that study the problems in menopause that women go through and seek for solutions. Let alone forming societies, men were completely silent about this issue. The mid-life crisis stories that came up one after another in the last two-three months gave [them] this opportunity.
> (Muftuoglu 2006a)

Muftuoglu considers the mid-life crisis stories as an opportunity to talk about andropause as a health issue, while highlighting his concern about the lack of attention paid to it. In addition, there is again the emphasis on how andropause should be framed differently from the mid-life crisis, even though the two can be seen in a patient at the same time.

Another crucial difference between menopause and andropause lies in the treatment approaches. Medical doctors are more cautious in advising hormone use in andropause compared to menopause. That may be partially attributed to the legacy of hormone treatments related to menopause (though in some examples both hormone treatments are advocated) and partially to the belief that andropause is not a universal experience like menopause. For instance, Professor Akkus, who is quoted above, answers the question 'Do you recommend hormone supplementation to men suffering from lack of testosterone, like menopausal women do?' as such:

> Not all of them. One has to think twice when giving hormones to men. Testosterone especially affects the prostate directly. It can trigger enlargement of the prostate gland or prostate cancer. Long-term treatments have side effects. It can negatively affect the liver and the nervous system.
>
> (*Hürriyet* 9 Aug. 2005)

In this logic, elucidated by an expert, vulnerability is attributed to men's bodies. Even though long-term hormone treatments can have negative effects on women's bodies as well, in the masculinist tone of talking about andropause, men are subject to higher standards of caution and anxiety. It is the men's bodies that should be protected.

'Azgın teke' syndrome: andropause as an excuse for marital infidelity

In the second category of news stories, andropause is portrayed as a social problem because it is seen as a reason for marital infidelity and crisis that may end with divorce. In this sense, andropause threatens and undermines the sacred social institution, the nuclear Turkish family, especially for the conservative-Islamist newspapers. The prototypical crisis portrayed is that the middle-aged man will start having a decrease in his libido and sexual performance, leading to a loss of self-confidence, and will cheat on his wife in an attempt to regain his masculine self-assurance and bravado. However, in most narratives the relation between loss of self-confidence and unfaithfulness is not fully questioned. It is considered as totally understandable that a man who has doubts about his sexuality would cheat on his wife and search for a younger, more attractive sex partner who can both challenge and prove his virility.

Several news stories in this category involve interviews with popular figures who had left their wives for younger women, and with their wives.

Examples include Halis Toprak, a major businessman; Neco, a pop singer; and Yasar Nuri Öztürk, a popular religious and political figure. One of the questions frequently asked of the wives is 'Do you think your husband did this because of andropause?' Attributing infidelity to a hormonal, medically accepted cause seems to be a tolerable and legitimate explanation. The question 'Are you in andropause?' is also asked of middle-aged men during interviews, sometimes regardless of whether they have issues with their wives or not. In this sense, we can say that the reporters or interviewers contribute to the narrative of andropause as a reason for mid-life crisis and infidelity by the frame they provide in these stories.

Some experts, when interviewed on the subject, make the connection between andropause and the search for a younger sex partner explicit:

> Prof. Sevuk, who emphasizes that men enter andropause after a certain age, stated that andropause is a psychological disorder despite the commonsensical belief that this disease does not affect sexuality. Attributing the condemnation of men in advanced ages who still feel young and are with younger women to the perspective of society, Dr Sevuk said 'Yet this relationship is completely normal. The societal judgments of "He is with a woman at his daughter's age, he is suffering from aging syndrome" has nothing to do with the sexuality of the man. There is also a psychological dimension for old men to be with young women. Young partner is the best aphrodisiac. When a man is with a much younger woman, his life view changes and his motivation and success increases.
>
> (Kunar 2002)

It is intriguing that here andropause is accepted as a psychological disorder rather than hormonal change or disturbance, while there is great tolerance (almost total legitimization and normalization) for aging men searching for younger sex partners. This psychologizing explanation is also used to explain marital infidelity and divorce cases in middle-aged couples. According to Dr Hattat, one of the most important self-claimed andrology experts of Turkey, 'andropause is a period when men cheat most'. Another public figure Dr Muftuoglu agrees with him in the same article and notes, 'Men in andropause stray more' (Muftuoglu 2006b).

Islamist-conservative newspapers and their columnists demonstrate greater anxiety over marital unfaithfulness and the possibility of divorce related to andropause and men's crisis more than the mainstream newspapers we surveyed. In *Zaman*, for example, one of the few articles on andropause listed its dangers, one of which was 'men divorcing their spouses and marrying younger women'. This was considered as 'perhaps the most dangerous' of the outcomes of a mid-life crisis/andropause, and was attributed to 'lack of strong bonds with the family' and 'lack of spiritual values' (Köseli 2010). It is very striking that this piece was the only one with a detectable critique of popular culture and the objectification of women related to andropause. The place of Islam – as one of the factors in marital infidelity due to andropause is rooted 'lack of spiritual values' – is also emphasized only by *Zaman* while mainstream-secular papers do not refer to religion in their narratives of andropause.

Insulting aging men: andropause as affront

In the final category of stories, andropause is used as an insult referring to mid-life crisis and aging. Aside from the *azgın teke* term explained above, which refers to the inappropriate sexual desires of aging men in mid-life crisis, columnists use it to demean rivals or popular figures, and politicians use it to criticize a rival party structure. An example of the former would be one columnist blaming another for being 'an andropausal man who turns love and women into kitsch with his theories' of understanding women (Turgut 2010). The implied meaning here is that an increased interest in women and relationships, and perhaps an unnecessary ambition to analyse these issues, is indicative of andropause.

The political element is slightly different from this meaning focused on love, sex and relationships with women. In 2009, at the height of *azgın teke* discussions in the magazine news, Sukru Ayalan, who was the deputy chairman of the ruling party (Justice and Development Party, JDP) at the time, accused the opposition party (Republican People's Party, RPP) of 'being ruled by administrators under menopause-andropause syndrome' (*Milliyet* 6 Oct. 2009). The context of his criticism was RPP's stubborn strategy of creating crisis and tension instead of coming up with solutions. Although this is a frequently pronounced criticism by ruling parties in general of the opposition party, backing up this trope with 'menopause-andropause syndrome' is a new strategy. Instead of a sexualized meaning, here the insult is more directed at the aging component of andropause, with the image of an old and stubborn person who does not want to change their ways and so harms those around him or her.

Conclusion

The politics of masculinities and the roles men might undertake in gendered intimacies in and outside the family became issues of social contestation not only in popular discourses but also in academic research and theoretical thinking in Turkey over the last decade (Özbay 2010a; Özbay *et al.* 2011; Sancar 2009). The media content we presented above points to a type of resistance to the tide of medicalization of the aging male body in popular narratives, through constructing andropause/male menopause as an excuse for impetuous (sexual) boyish mischief in the Turkish case. The hormonal portrayal of andropause in the medical discourse provides the basis for a more psychological explanation for mid-life crisis, which is characterized by the anxiety to prove virility and sexuality.

Despite the fact that narratives of andropause are often built upon the conceptualization of 'male menopause', aging male and female bodies are deemed and represented in quite different ways. The gendered construction of the aging female body invokes menopause, which involves an increase in responsibility on the woman's part to take care of herself, her body and her health, and make the right decisions while doing this (Erol 2009). Unlike the increased responsibilities for the menopausal woman, discourses around aging male bodies lead to a decrease in responsibility for men, creating a playful space in which men can have access to greater freedom, especially in terms of gender and sexual relations, as can be seen in the stories of marital infidelity justified, normalized and even encouraged with the instantiation of andropause. The health-related obligation to seek medical help and surveillance is still present in the andropause narratives of health columns and interviews with doctors. However, most advice depends on the existence of complaints defined around virility, mostly related to decreased energy or libido, rather than being about prevention as it is in the case of menopause. The difference between the menopause and andropause narratives is particularly striking given the 'universal', 'natural' and 'inevitable' character of menopause versus the 'individual', 'preventable' and 'trivialized' constructions of andropause.

In this context, hormones become *the* explanation for a psychological condition, in which middle-aged male subjects enact social misconduct and become negligent in their social and intimate relations. The counter-narrative for the tolerance shown to the 'boyish mischief' aspect of andropause comes in the form of shaming older men when they insist on acting like their younger counterparts. Similar to Wentzell's analysis of erectile dysfunction in relation to masculinity in older Mexican men (in this volume), there is an idea of 'age-appropriate masculinity' in the Turkish discourse of andropause, as demonstrated by the term *azgın teke*. However, although *azgın teke* is often reiterated as a derogatory term, and there is a narrative of shame around the stories on andropause and infidelity or seeking the company of younger women or sexual liaisons, these are referred through a language of tolerance and humour, if not permissiveness. These men are reprimanded at most; they are never expected to pay a real price for what they have done. Since sexual performance and virility are such important aspects of hegemonic Turkish masculinities (as elsewhere), anxieties around them become socially acceptable for aging men as well as their younger counterparts. Discourses of andropause haunt men from all generations and through the sarcastic and derisive tone applied, they thus serve to reinforce the existing gender inequality to the benefit of men in contemporary Turkey.

Notes

1 Connell's conceptualization of hegemonic masculinity have been criticized by many gender scholars in the last quarter century, see e.g. Seidler 2005. Connell

and Messerschmidt (2005) attempt to revise the concept in a response to these critics.
2 We tend to argue that the process in which men face with andropause in Turkey is characterized by the emotional politics of shame, as described by Ahmed: 'Shame can be described as an intense and painful sensation that is bound up with how the self feels about itself, a self-feeling that is felt by and on the body. … When shamed, one's body seems to burn up with the negation that is perceived (self-negation); and shame impresses upon the skin, as an intense feeling of the subject "being against itself"' (Ahmed 2004: 103)
3 There is an ongoing conflict between medical doctors in Turkey on defining andropause as a medical (and universal) condition or not. For example, Dr Aytug Kolankaya, a hugely popular obstetrics and gynaecology specialist who has a daily TV show called *Doktorum* (My Doctor), asserts: '[T]here is no medical condition called andropause. It is a psychological process that only some men at different ages pass through. It is not hormonal as it happens to women in menopause. Men start to ask existential questions of themselves, kind of a mid-life crisis at a certain age which depends on the person, and this mood affects his bodily mechanisms. It is not a medical condition that is seen in all male bodies. There are men over the age 70 and they have not entered andropause. It is possible.' (Personal communication)
4 Feminist writers across social sciences had documented men's gendered actions in relation to women before the year 2000 without incorporating theories and concepts of masculinity studies. See e.g. Kandiyoti 1994; Özbay 1990; Sirman 1990; Tekeli 1993.
5 We preferred to refer to the dictionary definitions of these two terms regarding male and female climacteric here rather than the (more nuanced and sometimes conflicting) medical definitions, since we are more interested in comparing the colloquial understandings of the terms for our analysis than in delving into the medical explanations.
6 The most famous example of these incidents involving celebrities happened around Neco, a famous male singer who was in his late 50s at the time, and known as a 'family guy'. He decided to divorce his wife of thirty years and married a much younger, 20-something woman. Neco and his previous wife had daughters older than the new wife. Nükhet Duru, a female pop-star and close friend of the now-divorced couple, sang an old, humorous song called *Kart Horoz* (The Old Cock) dedicated to Neco in front of TV cameras in order to criticize Neco's decision to leave his wife and children. She gave a voice to the hostile discourse against aged men who were irrationally and unresponsively searching for a fresh start, to a new life – how andropause is generally conceived in the Turkish popular discourses.

References

Ahmed, S. (2004) *The Politics of Emotion*, London: Routledge.
Aktas, F. O. (2009) 'Being a conscientious objector in Turkey: Challenging hegemonic masculinity in a militaristic nation-state', unpublished thesis, Central European University.
Atencio, M., and Koca, C. (2011) 'Gendered communities of practice and the construction of masculinities in Turkish physical education', *Gender and Education*, 23: 59–72.
Basaran, O. (2007) 'Militarized medicalized discourse on homosexuality and hegemonic masculinity in Turkey', unpublished thesis, Bogazici University.

Bereket, T., and Adam, B. D. (2006) 'The emergence of gay identities in contemporary Turkey', *Sexualities*, 9: 131–51.
Bilgin, E. (2004) 'An analysis of Turkish modernity through discourses of masculinities', unpublished dissertation, Middle East Technical University.
Bourke, J. (1996) *Dismembering the Male: Men's Bodies, Britain, and the Great War*, Chicago, IL: University of Chicago Press.
Broom, A. (2004) 'Prostate cancer and masculinity in Australian society: A case of stolen identity?', *International Journal of Men's Health*, 3(2): 73–91.
Connell, R. W. (1995) *Masculinities*, Berkeley, CA: University of California Press.
Connell, R. W. (2001) *The Men and the Boys*, Berkeley, CA: University of California Press.
Connell, R. W., and Messerschmidt, J. V. (2005) 'Hegemonic masculinity: Rethinking the concept', *Gender and Society*, 19(6): 829–59.
Conrad, P. (2007) *The Medicalization of Society: On the Transformation of Human Conditions into Treatable Disorders*, Baltimore, MD: Johns Hopkins University Press.
Courtenay, W. H. (2000) 'Constructions of masculinity and their influence on men's well-being: A theory of gender and health', *Social Science and Medicine*, 50(10): 1385–1401.
Delice, S. (2010) 'Friendship, sociability, and masculinity in the Ottoman Empire: An essay confronting the ghosts of historicism', *New Perspectives on Turkey*, 42: 103–25.
Duman, S. (2006) 'Azgın Teke Sendromu', *Vatan* (23 Sept.).
Ehrkamp, P. (2008) 'Risking publicity: Masculinities and the racialization of public neighborhood space', *Social and Cultural Geography*, 9: 117–33.
Erol, M. (2003) 'İktidar, Teknoloji ve Maskulinite', unpublished thesis, Yildiz Technical University.
Erol, M. (2009) 'Tales of the second spring: Menopause in Turkey through the narratives of menopausal women and gynecologists', *Medical Anthropology*, 28: 368–96.
Ersan, M. (2005) 'Erkeklerin yarısı menopozu hiç duymamış, kadın-erkek andropozu duymayanlar ise yarıdan daha fazla', *Hürriyet* (9 Aug.).
Ewing, K. P. (2008) *Stolen Honor: Stigmatizing Muslim Men in Berlin*, Stanford, CA: Stanford University Press.
Gerschick, J. T., and Miller, A. S. (1994) 'Coming to terms: Masculinity and physical disability', *Masculinities*, 2(1): 34–55.
Guillemin, M. (2000) 'Working practices of the menopause clinic', *Science, Technology, and Human Values*, 25(4): 449–71.
Houck, J. A. (2006) *Hot and Bothered: Women, Medicine, and Menopause in Modern America*, Cambridge, MA: Harvard University Press.
Inhorn, M. C. (1994) *Quest for Conception: Gender, Fertility, and Egyptian Medical Traditions*, Philadelphia, PA: University of Pennsylvania Press.
Kandiyoti, D. (1994) 'The paradoxes of masculinity: Some thoughts on segregated societies', in A. Cornwall and N. Lindisfarne (eds), *Dislocating Masculinity: Comparative Ethnographies* (pp. 197–212), London: Routledge.
Kartal, A. (1997) 'Öteki kadın operasyonu', *Hürriyet* (21 Aug.).
Kunar, S. (2002) 'Yaşlı erkeklere genç sevgili dopingi', *Hürriyet* (21 Oct.).
Kimmel, M. (2009) *Guyland: The Perilous World Where Boys Become Men*, New York: Harper.

Kizilkan, N. (2009) 'Spaces of masculinities: Bachelor rooms in Suleymaniye', unpublished thesis, Middle East Technical University.
Köseli, B. (2010) 'Kırk yaşıma geldim sendromlardayım', *Zaman* (4 July).
Lock, M. (1993) *Encounters with Aging: Mythologies of Menopause in Japan and North America*, Berkeley and Los Angeles, CA: University of California Press.
Loe, M. (2004) *The Rise of Viagra: How the Little Blue Pill Changed Sex in America*, New York: New York University Press.
McDowell, L. (2003) *Redundant Masculinities: Employment Change and White Working Class Youth*, Oxford: Blackwell.
Marshall, B. L. (2006) 'The new virility: Viagra, male aging and sexual function', *Sexualities*, 9: 345–62.
Marshall, B. L. (2007) 'Climacteric redux? (Re)medicalizing the male menopause', *Men and Masculinities*, 9: 509–29.
Marshall, B. L. (2009) 'Constructing the "aging male": Negotiating sameness and difference in biomedical accounts of menopause and andropause', paper presented at Society for the Social Study of Science (4S) Annual Meetings, Crystal City, VA, Oct.
Martin, E. (1987) *The Woman in the Body: A Cultural Analysis of Reproduction*, Boston, MA: Beacon Press.
Messner, M. (1997) *Politics of Masculinities: Men in Movements*, Lanham, MD: AltaMira.
Milliyet (2009) 'AKPli vekil belden aşağı vurdu', *Milliyet* (10 June).
Muftuoglu, O. (2006a) 'Andropoz Fırtınası', *Hürriyet* (25 Sept.).
Muftuoglu, O. (2006b) 'Andropozdaki Erkek Daha Çok Aldatıyor', *Hürriyet* (21 Sept.).
Oliffe, J. (2005) 'Constructions of masculinity following prostatectomy-induced impotence', *Social Science and Medicine*, 60(10): 2249–59.
Oudshoorn, N. (1997) 'Menopause, only for women? The social construction of menopause as an exclusively female condition', *Journal of Psychosomatic Obstetrics and Gyneacology*, 18: 137–44.
Özbay, C. (2010a) 'Neoliberalizm ve Erkeklik Halleri', in A. Ozturk (ed.), *Yeni Sol, Yeni Sag* (pp. 645–663), Ankara: Phoenix.
Özbay, C. (2010b) 'Nocturnal queers: Rent boys' masculinity in Istanbul', *Sexualities*, 13(5): 645–63.
Özbay, C., Terzioglu, A., and Yasin, Y. (eds) (2011) *Neoliberalizm ve Mahremiyet: Turkiye'de Beden, Saglik ve Cinsellik*, Istanbul: Metis.
Özbay, F. (1990) *Women, Family and Social Change*, Bangkok: UNESCO.
Rosenfeld, D., and Faircloth, C. A. (2006) 'Introduction: Medicalized masculinities. The missing link?', in D. Rosenfeld and C. A. Faircloth (eds), *Medicalized Masculinities* (pp. 1–20), Philadelphia, PA: Temple University Press.
Rothman, B. K. (1989) *Recreating Motherhood: Ideology and Technology in a Patriarchal Society*, New York: Norton.
Sabo, D. (2005) 'The study of masculinities and men's health: An overview', in M. S. Kimmel, J. Hearn, and R. W. Connell (eds), *Handbook of Studies on Men and Masculinities* (pp. 326–352), London: Sage.
Sabo, D., and Gordon, D. F. (eds) (1995) *Men's Health and Illness: Gender, Power, and the Body*, London: Sage.
Sancar, S. (2009) *Erkeklik: Imkansiz Iktidar*, Istanbul: Metis.

Seidler, V. J. (2005) *Transforming Masculinities: Men, Cultures, Bodies, Power, Sex and Love*, London: Routledge.
Sinclair-Webb, E. (2006) 'Our Bulent is a commando: Military service and manhood in Turkey', in M. Ghoussoub and E. Sinclair-Webb (eds), *Imagined Masculinities: Male Identity and Culture in the Modern Middle East* (pp. 65–102), London: Saqi.
Sirman, N. (1990) 'State, village and gender in Western Turkey', in A. Finkel and N. Sirman (eds), *Turkish State, Turkish Society* (pp. 21–52), London: Routledge.
Sokmen, S. (ed.) (2004) 'Erkeklik', *Toplum and Bilim*, 101, Istanbul: Birikim.
Szymczak, J. E., and Conrad, P. (2006) 'Medicalizing the aging male body: Andropause and baldness', in D. Rosenfeld and C. A. Faircloth (eds), *Medicalized Masculinities* (pp. 89–111), Philadelphia, PA: Temple University Press.
Tekeli, S. (ed.) (1993) *1980'ler Turkiye'sinde Kadin Bakis Acisindan Kadinlar*, Istanbul: Iletisim.
Turgut, S. (2010) 'Andropoz Erkekleri', *Akşam* (14 Feb.).
Watkins, E. S. (2007a) *The Estrogen Elixir: A History of Hormone Replacement Therapy in America*, Baltimore, MD: Johns Hopkins University Press.
Watkins, E. S. (2007b) 'The medicalisation of male menopause in America', *Social History of Medicine*, 20(2): 369–88.
Wienke, C. (2006) 'Sex the natural way: The marketing of Cialis and Levitra', in D. Rosenfeld and C. A. Faircloth (eds), *Medicalized Masculinities* (pp. 45–64), Philadelphia, PA: Temple University Press.

Part IV
Care work

10 Older men

The health and caring paradox

Kate Davidson

Introduction

Throughout their life course, men tend to have an ambivalent relationship with health and illness, both their own and that of other people. Running parallel to this ambivalence is men's attitude to caring and being cared for, which can be viewed as an assault on their manhood. This chapter examines the health and caring paradox experienced by older men. Men, young and old, face significant challenges when dealing with both chronic and life-threatening illness, but it is primarily in later life that they face the challenge of coping with the necessity of caring for a sick loved one, usually a spouse. Oftentimes these older men have health issues themselves and so experience a 'double whammy' realignment of their sense of manliness. The chapter comprises three main sections. First it will offer a brief review of the literature on masculinity and health in old age. Only comparatively recently has there been interest shown in older men's subjectivity of waning strength and power owing to failing health and loss of status in a youth orientated global culture. Second it outlines the methods and results of data analysis from three qualitative research projects carried out in the United Kingdom between 1995 and 2005.[1] In total, 151 men over the age of 65 and living independently in the community were interviewed. Not all these men were in poor health, not all were being cared for by their spouse or another; nor were all undertaking care of a loved one, but all discussed their health and its impact on their identity as old men. Third this chapter discusses the findings from these three projects. The data revealed that for these men, whether ill or well, caring or cared for, alone or with a partner, their sense of manhood was undiminished but altered to 'best fit' their current lived experience. We conclude that, despite increasing physical frailties when their bodies are 'letting them down', these older men called on their sense of manhood, resilience and stoicism to negotiate and define their experience of aging. The chapter draws substantially on previous publications by the author and her colleagues,[2] to whom she is grateful for their permission to make use of relevant parts of these publications. The publications either focused on 'older men and health' or 'older men and caring'. What is new here is the melding of the older men's attitude to health and their experience of caring and being cared for, in an attempt to do justice to the rich complexity and contradictions of real, struggling men.

Masculinity, health and aging

Within contemporary Western societies, the dominant, hegemonic ideology is said to prioritize such traits as physical strength, virility, wealth, self-control and aggression (Petersen 1998). It is also said to prioritise youth (Whitehead 2002). Connell (2000) suggests that there are multiple masculinities, which coexist in time and space and which compete for dominance. Of particular note here is hegemonic masculinity or the dominant, most 'honoured or desired' form of masculinity as discussed elsewhere in this volume. As men age, their withdrawal from the occupational 'breadwinner' role, possible loss of sexual potency, diminishing physical strength and the onset of illness can all weaken their relationship with this dominant ideology (Arber *et al.* 2003). During the 1990s, scholars suggested that 'men's health is profoundly affected by power differences that shape relationships between men and women, women and women, and men and men' (Sabo 2005: 328). Courtney (1998, 2000) and Cameron and Bernardes (1998) for example, identified how men see health as women's business and responsibility. They argued that men know little about men's health; men tend to keep quiet about their health problems; they tend to deny themselves a self-monitoring role (as health promotion is 'female'); men cope less well because of a fear of losing control and they tend to delay seeking help. These social practices which undermine men's health were considered tools used to approximate hegemonic masculine ideals and to negate the (idealized) feminine norms of health care utilization and positive health beliefs. In essence, 'doing health' was identified as a form of 'doing gender' (Saltonstall 1993: 12).

Robertson (2003) challenges what he considers to be a somewhat simplistic, deterministic gendered approach. He suggests that men face a dilemma between showing they do not care and realizing that they should care, which he terms the *should care/don't care* dichotomy and, as a result, caring for health needs to be *legitimized* or explained in some way by men. On the one hand, 'real' men are strong, indestructible and in control of their lives, including risk-taking and indulging in unhealthy practices such as smoking and unsafe alcohol consumption. On the other hand, men feel the need to look after their bodies in order to maintain their employment status or pursue a sport activity or provide for a family, or all three. Gough (2006: 2486) also highlights how some men may 'have access to resources which enable "healthy" reinvention of identities and practices while remaining complicit with hegemonic ideals'. Moynihan (1998) observed in her research on young males with testicular cancer that the men found it hard to accept being ill. Taking their condition 'like a man' meant hiding behind a brave face and refusing to express their fears and needs. She argues that the way the doctor deals with the 'sick man', and the language used in explanation of a condition (and its consequences), allows the patient to maintain a sense of masculinity. For example, male clinicians used such metaphors as 'a plane flying on one engine and landing safely' or that 'one cylinder is as good as two' (ibid. 1074). Men tend to take a mechanistic view of their bodies, as controllable, and controlled. Indeed, as Seidler (1994) points out, this highlights the Cartesian duality of mind and body, where men separate their physical and emotional existences. However, within her study of older adult's experience of Parkinson disease, Solimeo (2008) highlights the importance of role continuity in later life. This may be especially difficult for those men who do not have the physical or economic resources available to them or those men who damaged their health in earlier pursuit of hegemonic masculinities (Calasanti and King 2005).

Thompson (1994) identifies a divide within the gerontological literature between those who believe that old men are emasculated by aging and those who suggest that old men may have to adapt to fit into a new, but not substantially different, dominant ideological form of masculinity as they age. The assumption within both schools of thought is that manhood is constructed 'through and by reference to "age"' (Hearn 1995: 97), and that a sense of maleness is defined and redefined throughout the life course. Therefore, a life-course approach allows for investigation into how life transitions affect the relationship between masculinities, health and embodied experience. Delay in seeking help, McVittie and Willcock (2006) argue, is not simply explained by stoicism which characterizes hegemonic masculinity. Although identities of being a 'real man' and a 'healthy man' are not easily relinquished, age and life experience bring about the negotiation of different forms of masculine identities. Some academics who have been involved with young men and masculinities for many years are now beginning to address their own aging bodies. For example, Jackson wrote about macho values and adolescent boys (Salisbury and Jackson 1996). In his critical autobiographical project Jackson (2003) recognizes that, as he ages, there are multi-dimensional and counter-hegemonic models of masculinity which have developed in him a more reintegrated acceptance of himself and his life:

> A new language of how to be a different kind of man has come along with my processes of ageing and bodily disruptions and emotional transitions. ... Neither do I negatively measure my embodied self against the idealised norms of hegemonic masculinity any more.
> (Jackson 2003: 86)

Jackson's reflection echoes the excellent discussion on age and embodiment in the Third and Fourth Ages by Higgs and McGowan in this volume.

It has been suggested that it is not just aging that triggers realignment of masculine discourses (Meadows and Davidson 2006). Events such as marriage and fatherhood may (unconsciously) draw men 'towards responsible conviviality' (Mullen 1993: 177, quoted in Watson 2000: 39) and the successful balancing of control and release or moderation and excess. Somewhat similarly, it is well documented in successive UK General Household Surveys that older married men report better health than widowed, divorced or never married men (Davidson and Arber 2003). At all ages over 50, divorced and separated men, followed by widowed men, report poorer health than single or married/cohabiting men (Thomas *et al.* 1998). Divorced men over the age of 50 report higher rates of smoking and hazardous alcohol intake than other men of their age (Davidson and Arber 2003) and solo living in old age is associated with an increased likelihood of experiencing loneliness, social isolation and depression (Victor *et al.* 2002). The maintenance of masculinity in an alien (dependent and feminized) environment is germane to their selfhood, and is negotiated in order to 'best fit' their altered circumstances (Davidson and Meadows 2010). The following section reports three research projects carried out by the author and her colleagues at the Centre for Research on Ageing and Gender at the University of Surrey, UK.

The research projects

The three research projects that provide the data for this chapter were very diverse in scale and methodologies. However, they each contained a component of qualitative, in-depth interviews with men between the ages of 65 and 91, living independently in the community. The average age of the participants was 75 years. A total of 151 men were interviewed, of whom 50 were married/cohabiting, 74 widowed, 12 divorced/separated and 15 never married (all names are anonymized to protect confidentiality). The divorced/separated men were the youngest group, with an average age of 68, and there were none over the age of 76. This contrasts with the oldest group, the widowers, whose average age was 79: 29 out of 74 were 80 plus, with only 6 under 70. A few of the partnership histories of the older men interviewed were complex. For example, some men had been married more than once: some had been divorced and then widowed, and some had been widowed or divorced and were now cohabiting. For the analysis, the men were categorized by their current partnership status. The over-representation of men without partners reflected the research rationale in each project, which sought to study older men who lived alone. The samples were recruited through a variety of avenues including general practitioners' registers, faith groups and establishments, military, sports and leisure clubs, day centres, a senior community, voluntary organizations and 'word of mouth' of colleagues and their relatives.

A vital aspect of the sample is worth noting here. All the men were white and most had enjoyed years of stable, or serial-continuous employment, some having achieved well-paid and high-status careers, even from quite modest beginnings. The sample consequently comprised relatively privileged men who had benefited from the prosperity resulting from post World War II UK social, economic and welfare state improvements. They were self-selected, articulate and highly motivated to contribute to the three studies. We are mindful that a major limitation of our work is the lack of voice of men who were openly homosexual, although one never married participant did admit 'I suppose I was what they call "gay" now. But I never did anything about it.' A committed Christian, he lived with his mother after she was widowed and cared for her during her later years. Nor did we interview ethnic-minority older men (who did not volunteer, despite concentrated contact with faith groups), those who were socially and economically deprived or those with severe mental and physical health problems, again because there was no response from these groups to our recruitment drive. The research protocols meant that we interviewed no men with Alzheimer's disease or dementia.

For the three projects we used software programmes for computer-assisted qualitative data analysis (WinMax pro, NVivo and MAXqda respectively). Similar strategies were employed for text coding and theme building, memo making and data retrieval that meant we were able to maintain a robust comparison between the projects. The analyses were based on the grounded theory perspective (Strauss and Corbin 2008) that permits the percolation of pertinent themes through the data. Utilizing iterative, interpretive and reflexive processes (Mason 1996a), we constructed explanations and arguments to address our intellectual puzzle: what is it like to be a man and get old? Although the analyses were carried out by different research assistants the author was strategically involved with all the studies and oversaw the procedures.

We took a life-course approach which enabled investigation into how 'the self of the past is the underpinning of the self of the present' (Thompson and Whearty 2004: 8). In the UK, for example, a man with a history of working in a professional occupation and living in south-east England, is likely to outlive his unskilled manual compatriot in Scotland by some twelve years, with a projected life expectancy of 83 years compared to 71 years (StatBase 2002; Emslie *et al.* 2004). However, a life-course perspective needs to be balanced by an appreciation of cohort effects (Goldscheier 1990). The vast majority of the men served within the British Forces at some point in their lives, either during the hostilities of the Second World War, or during conscription that lasted in the UK until 1960. The military environment was an almost exclusively male domain, and there it was imperative to assert their masculinity in order to distance themselves from both femininity and homosexuality (Segal 1990). What was considered appropriate masculine behaviour was reinforced through traditions and customs within military life. The men also had experienced some degree of discipline, self-discipline and deprivation of personal freedom and to some extent could call on these 'reserves' in later life when faced with challenges to their autonomy and sense of control.

Health matters

A common thread through all the interview schedules was their health status, attitudes to health professionals and health promoting practices. What emerged from the qualitative analysis was a complex picture of health awareness, protection strategies and risk-taking. Our interviews with the older men revealed that they knew what was 'good' and what was 'bad' for healthy living. This does not necessarily mean that the men simply put this knowledge into practice. Rather, a system of checks and balances or 'trade offs' evolved for most of the men. The direct quotes are prefixed by a fictitious name, the respondent's age and marital status. The individual research project is not identified in the interest of simplicity.

> Jon (72, married): I should walk more. I suppose if I walk round to the post box round the corner, that's the furthest I go during the week. We try and walk at weekends. I'm a bad lad I know. Like for breakfast, I will get up in the morning and probably have two pots of tea, bad for you, eight cups of tea, eight spoonfuls of sugar – wrong. It used to be sixteen, but I have cut the sugar down. Lunch I might have a cheese sandwich, bad for me again. But then I have an evening meal. It would be a cooked meal. Last night it was bacon, tonight it will be a small roast. ... I like a drink, I probably drink too much, more than what I should do.

Weather permitting, Jon and his wife went for long afternoon walks at the weekend by way of compensation for taking little exercise during the week. Jon was not alone in compensating for risky health behaviours. Several said they rarely drank alcohol on Mondays because they would have had several drinks over the weekend. Some only ever drank alcohol at weekends, or if they were in company, but felt that because they had abstained they could 'indulge' themselves more when they did.

Very few of the men admitted to being 'dangerous' drinkers; that is, more than 50 units of alcohol a week. One was a divorced man who drank wine steadily throughout the interview and offered the interviewer a glass. It was 11 am. However, as mentioned above, the men monitored their drinking, generally keeping it to weekends and when in company. The married men drank more regularly, often having a drink with their wife before and at dinner. Like Jon above, a few commented that they probably drank near or over the recommended weekly limit of 28 units. The widowed and single men drank the least often, and it was the divorced men, although not all, who tended to be either abstainers (two were recovering alcoholics) or heavy drinkers.

Most of the men had smoked when younger, and only five (all divorced) continued to smoke more than 40 cigarettes a day. Some of the married men admitted to having a cigar 'on high days and holidays' but most had either ceased, or dramatically cut down their smoking. Interestingly, those who continued to have the occasional cigarette did so in the garden 'because she [their wife] doesn't like the smell in the house'. This could reflect changing societal attitudes to smoking but also may reflect the wife's disapproval of smoking. Those who had given up or cut down when they were younger tended to do so for economic reasons: taking on a mortgage, having children and so on. Those who gave up in later years tended to do it for health reasons, and usually on 'doctor's orders'. One gave up after his wife died of cancer, and his daughter had begged him to stop.

These older men's narratives resonate with Robertson's (2006) work on younger men. He suggests (ibid. 178) that younger men have to manage two conflicting discourses: 'first that "real" men do not care about health and second, that the pursuit of health is a moral requirement for good citizenship'. Further:

> it is not just caring too much about health that puts hegemonic identity at risk. Not to take enough care with one's health, particularly through indulging in excess, also moves one away from hegemonic ideals. It suggests irresponsibility and lack of control, which then becomes representative of transgressive (male) behaviour.
> (Robertson 2006: 184)

Similar to the younger men in Robertson's study, the older men here appear embroiled in a should care/don't care balancing act and are required to tread a path between control and release. For some, the ability to achieve this balancing act later in life seemed worth emphasizing; suggesting that it may take on greater importance in situations where other tools and resources used to approximate hegemonic forms of masculinity are not available. This was demonstrated in how some men perceived their control over their bodies and their health:

> Rory (84, married): I'm one of these lucky people that have suffered good health all my life. ... we are sensible about our eating, we try and do a certain amount of walking exercise each day.

> Peter (70, widowed): I have been wonderfully fit, apart from back trouble since my wife died. I don't drink lots of alcohol, I don't smoke, I live a fairly simple lifestyle, a healthy lifestyle.

For many of the men, it was apparent that 'control' literally meant '*self-control*' and that this, in turn, meant that the men rarely engaged with professional preventive health programmes. Good citizenship meant taking responsibility for one's health, and self-discipline a way of achieving it without medical intervention.

Men and health professionals

It is a common observation that men have a different relationship with health professionals than do women (Lee and Owens 2002). Women have a more health-related relationship – contraception, pregnancy, child immunization and developmental checks, and their own health screening – consequently the step to illness consultation is short. On the other hand, men's relationship is somewhat one-dimensional – that is, sickness orientated. When they eventually consult a health professional, it is possible they will hear the bad news they have been postponing (Davidson and Arber 2003). This difference, however, is seen as a weakness in women, and a strength for men.

> Jon (72, married): I think it is like, well, ladies will go to the doctors many, many times more than a man. A man says – oh, it came by itself, it will go by itself.

We asked the men about their contact with the medical profession. Common to each partnership status were men who said they seldom went to their GP surgery. We categorized these men into 'sceptics' and 'stoics'.

When talking about the medical profession, the sceptics used phrases like: 'most of them are a waste of time', one said: 'I don't like doctors, I keep as far away from the place ... it's not an exact science', and went on to say that meteorology and medicine were about as accurate as each other. Another said that he would rather go to a veterinary surgeon than a doctor. The stoics on the other hand said things like:

> Gareth (71, widowed): ... a lot of illnesses, people can deal with it themselves.

> Paul (67, divorced): I don't give in. Even if I felt awful, I wouldn't tell anyone.

> Richard (70, never married): I've always tended to think, well, it's going to go away.

> Edward (71, never married): You've just got to get through it.

However, there was a surprisingly high reportage of asthma for which the men were prescribed an inhaler. Similarly, men reported taking medication for high blood pressure. There were a number of men who had undergone major treatment/surgery and saw their physician for regular check-ups – from quarterly to biennially: 'you have to see them once a year, and he sort of puts the old stethoscope on, asks a few questions and tells you to come back next year'. The men who reported these routine compliance visits did not see them as 'sickness' consultations and, interestingly, tended not count them as 'going to the doctor', until the interviewer probed. That is, the men said they rarely went to their general practitioner (GP) surgery when originally asked, and then later disclosed a longer term condition which required regular follow up health visits and/or repeat prescriptions. Compliance visits, as opposed to those which were self-initiated, did not seem to 'register'. Thus the men were able to maintain their notion of appropriate masculine behaviour, as they constructed frequent use of health care as feminine and infrequent use as normal.

> Andrew (72, widowed): My neighbour is always at the surgery with something or other and she's bothering the GP who should be tending to people who are really ill.

Andrew is simultaneously constructing help-seeking behaviours as negative (bothering GPs) and female. The 'frequent use of health care = female' vs 'the seldom user of health care = male' construction can conflict with the men's attempts to perform 'the should care/don't care' balancing act (Robertson, 2006). As Noone and Stephens (2008) identify in their interview study of seven older men, a third subject position exists which enables men to resolve this dilemma and use health care while maintaining a masculine identity. They label this the 'legitimate user position', when men stress that they do not go running to the doctor for everything.

Within the three studies, the 'legitimate user position' was intrinsically linked to marital status. For example, Jess offered the following:

> Jess (71, married): My wife has her 'woman' checks. She said to me 'If I've got to do this, why don't you too?', so I do, just to keep her happy. She says she wants me to be around a long time!

Jess echoed the comments from several men who joked that their wives nagged them to go to the GP because they wanted them to be fit and healthy. They also said things like 'she'll only get on at me if I don't'. As White (2001: 19) argues, 'when a man is ill it is normally the female member of the family ... who sanctions the illness behaviour'. Although this can be a means of legitimizing visits to a doctor, it paradoxically reinforces the notion that health care is women's concern. Again, however, this compliance to a wife's 'nagging' helps sustain a sense of manliness as they can justify help seeking only because they have been prompted.

Unsurprisingly, the older the man, the more likely he was to have increased contact with health professionals. About a third of the men in the studies reported very poor health and frequent contact with health professionals. Most of these men had been ill for several years, some had undergone extensive surgery and many of these were taking a 'veritable medicine chest' of prescription drugs. Some said that they had been 'fine' until they went to the doctor with one complaint, and then all sorts of other medical conditions were diagnosed. Interestingly, it was more often widowers who reported this. Almost invariably, they had waited until their wife died before consulting a doctor, many ignoring symptoms of illness, as they could not afford to be sick while they were caring for her. In the meantime, the conditions were stacking up. We termed these 'domino pathologies' – they went with one condition and came out with several (Davidson and Arber 2003).

> Forrest (widowed): I'm now 81 and I'm in poor health, very poor health. Up until the age of 75, just after my wife died, I was going fine and then I had a serious cancer operation. After that, everything seemed to break down.

The older the man, the closer the dominos and the quicker the tumble into multiple conditions. A life-course history of denial is ingrained, but doctor avoidance becomes a vicious circle. Many of the men interviewed admitted to postponing making an appointment until they were very sick. They then have negative associations with the doctor, who they see when they are in pain, or feel very unwell and, importantly, who may give them bad news about their health. Whatever pathway was travelled to get professional help, many of the participants felt that going to the doctor in the first place was the start of their deterioration in health, rather than identification of pre-existing conditions.

Although women live longer than men on average, they have a higher morbidity (Lee and Owens 2002). Men in higher socio-economic groups tend to survive longer into old age and tend to report good subjective health (Arber and Cooper 1999) and are more likely than younger married men to care for an ailing spouse with chronic disease (Ribeiro and Paul 2008).

Older men and caring: the paradox

It was taken for granted that, assuming she was not ill or predeceased him, a married man would be looked after by his wife in the case of failing health and as such was not a major issue in the interviews. The fear of becoming a burden was more likely to be explicitly expressed by the older widowers than the older divorced and never married men. Divorced and never married men were also concerned about deteriorating health but were less likely to mention the possibility of being cared for by an adult relative, either because none was available, or they did not have the sort of relationship they could fall back on when the need arose. For the never married men in particular there was an underlying assumption that if they were very ill, one day they might 'have to go into a home' which reflects a long-term understanding that they were without a close family network in their later years.

Anthony Giddens's (1994) analysis of ontological security of the self in late modernity resonates with the self-construct in a realignment of the meaning of self-identity following a major life change, such as caring, or being dependent on another for care. He argues that confidence in daily life and the sustenance of an adequate narrative of self-identity is maintained through a sense of ontological security. Davidson *et al.* (2000) concluded that in a marital relationship, regardless of whether an older man was cared for by his wife, or he was the one who cared, he maintained a sense of self as 'head of the household' and retained more control within the marital home. Calasanti (2003: 22) suggests that men adopt a managerial style to care work that enables them to separate 'caring for' and 'caring about'. The men in these studies negotiated and realigned their masculinity within the feminized domain of caring. They combated the potentially negative connotations of loss of manhood by defining their care responsibilities in organizational, instrumental and functional terms.

> Darren (82, widowed): I got a nurse to come in to bathe her on occasion, weekly or whatever it was ... but the rest I did myself. Yes, I looked after her all the time. Just like doing another job, except indoors!

> Tom (76, widowed): I used to do all the cooking and all that sort of thing. I did everything for her. I'd get her up in the morning, wash her, dress her. I used to have to put her bra on and everything. Then I'd wash her hair, put curlers in, take out. No particular style just tidy. I got a good sort of routine, you just have to be organized.

Only one married participant, George (66), reported that he was undertaking full-time care of his wife who suffered from multiple sclerosis. He had promised her before she became severely debilitated that she would never go into residential care. When she could no longer look after herself he converted the garage into what he described as the 'hospital wing'. He then employed a care agency to come in daily, including weekends, and carry out personal hygiene routines. As she deteriorated further, he employed an agency to come in overnight. This meant he could have 'a semblance of a normal life' to carry out his duties as a Freemason Lodge Officer. He was proud that he had kept his promise (caring about), had organized people to look after her (caring for) and continued to maintain a standing in the community (masculine identity). There were of course several periods of the day that he was alone with her but it was interesting that his perception of full-time care did not conflate with the criteria that Darren and Tom above set themselves. However, George was one of the youngest participants and was still in employment when his wife first needed increased care. He was also economically secure and was able to organize and pay for her care.

Many of the men who cared for an ailing wife reported that friends, family and health professionals 'didn't know how they coped'. Gus (82, widowed), for example, talks about how his reply to a nurse who said 'We are worried about you, you know' was to categorically state 'No, I will carry on'. Rose and Bruce (1995) point out that, in a society which considers elderly male spouse carers to be 'Mr Wonderful', the assistance they receive from professional health and welfare workers and the esteem in which they are held differs greatly from that offered to and accorded to women. In their study, Rose and Bruce found themselves, as committed feminists, driving home from interviews with older male carers saying to each other 'What a wonderful man':

> Reproducing Mr Wonderful was all too easy, but to reproduce such an undifferentiated and stereotypically positive picture of the women carers was not, for we had not been given such an account. Instead women had offered us a less positive, more nuanced, account of the diversity among women, for whom care giving was nonetheless an expected activity.
> (Rose and Bruce 1995: 127)

Mason (1996b) took the argument further by distinguishing between 'active sensibility' and 'sentient activity'. Active sensibility, she argues, operates on a conscious plane in terms of physical care activities and decision-making in relation to performing tasks and is therefore highly visible. Sentient activity, on the other hand, operates on a less conscious plane, often carried out on 'auto pilot' from long-term experience and entails consideration for another, sensitivity to likes and dislikes learned over time. This activity is largely invisible and almost always taken for granted. Whilst by no means discretely gendered, the former relates more to men and their organizational strategies and their sense of 'another career' that has to be carried out to the best of their ability. Even so, denial of the gravity of a wife's condition may mean the care was not always appropriate:

> Barry (78, widowed): I always took the attitude 'Now come on, come on. We've got to have a strong mind about this, you know. We're going to beat this cancer.' But I always wonder whether I should have talked more to her about dying and all the things that you don't know until you do. But I have no guilt; I have no guilt, because whatever I did, I did. I have no guilt.

Barry copes with his reflection on his behaviour by convincing himself he did the 'right thing at the time' and so does not blame himself.

The complexities involved with men's constructions of health and health care utilization, the balancing of masculine identities and the moral requirement to be good citizens did find some of the men literally in 'no man's land'. The physical decline described some of the men provoked critical reflection on their lives in a way that reflects Jackson's (1990) discussion of how his bodily breakdown enabled him to 'legitimately' take up an alternative masculinity.

Sean (72, married): I have done a lot of silly things because I was very headstrong at that time too. I was very much in control of the family, but I have learned to be – I have allowed myself to be trodden on once a while, and it seems to work better.

Here, Sean's insight illustrates an acceptance of alternative ways of dealing with his manliness, and although he associates relinquishing control with being trodden on, he admits that life seems to be easier when you 'give in'. He sighed deeply.

Conclusion

Although we did not interview men who had mental health problems, we did interview men who cared for a wife with dementia or Alzheimer's, and our findings resonate very much with those of Kimmel and Coston in this volume. However, we consider our research has led to a better understanding of the differentiation of older men according to *partnership* status. Older men who are divorced are a growing segment of the population, but were found to be significantly disadvantaged in terms of their higher levels of health-risk behaviours, particularly smoking and drinking. Older lone men in particular, are less likely to have a caretaker to monitor their health behaviours, or a gatekeeper to encourage health consultation – they lack the 'nag and drag' scenario (personal communication).

When asked about diet, physical activity, smoking and alcohol consumption, all the men were aware of what was 'good' for them, and the likelihood of ill health resulting from risk behaviours. These attitudes reflect Robertson's (2003) should care/don't care balance. We could surmise that older men are aware of health promotion information, but, similar to other groups in society, they do not always adhere to advice. However, for the population of older men, the results of ignoring such advice can be more devastating than for younger generations, given that men continue to be at higher risk of catastrophic ill health earlier than women.

For men who have had little or no 'ongoing contact' with health professionals (unlike women) in their life course, it seems unlikely that they will turn to health professionals when they reach later life. Whilst women have routinely visited the doctor through the life course, for family planning, pregnancy, or to take their children for clinics, immunization programmes as well as when they are sick, the men in this study seemed to consider going to the doctor as a sign of weakness. 'I think it is like, well, ladies will go to the doctors many, many times more than a man. A man says – oh, it came by itself, it will go by itself.' They did not want to be seen to 'give in' to sickness. It is important to recognize that the customary approach to health improvement has been to target individuals, but less attention has been paid to addressing the broad determinants of older men's health behaviours. These include biological, social, cultural and economic factors in influencing men's choices of health protective strategies.

The men who (had) cared for their wife were able to find alternative models of masculinity which permitted them to maintain a sense of manliness by setting up strategies of organization and management of their alien circumstance, akin to their earlier life experience. In doing so, they attract praise and admiration in the public sphere which offsets the new private career.

The key achievements of these research projects have been to demonstrate how masculinity continues to structure men's experiences in late life, despite onset of ill health, the need to care for a spouse, widowhood or living alone. We sought to examine their lives beyond biological differences between men and women, and through taking a life-course approach with our in-depth interviews, investigate the socially constructed roles that have shaped and manipulated their sense of masculinity to 'best fit' their altered lives and changing bodies. We conclude that these older men felt no less of a man than they did in their virile youth, but viewed the passing of that part of their lives with pragmatism and regret rather than anger.

There are still many gaps in our understanding of older men's experience of aging bodies and minds and the compensatory elasticity employed in coming to terms with altered masculine identities. Second wave feminists of the 1970s began to conceptualize growing old as women, and it is timely that men who have devoted years of academic endeavour in getting to grips with younger men's essence of themselves should start telling us how it is for them in the second decade of the twnty-first century. This chapter pushes on an open door.

Notes

1 K. Davidson, 'Gender, age and widowhood: How older widows and widowers differently realign their lives', unpublished thesis, University of Surrey, UK, 1999. S. Arber and K. Davidson, 'The social worlds and health behaviours of older men' (1999–2002), funded by the Economic and Social Research Council (ESRC)– Grant no. L480 25 4033. Food in Later Life project (2003–5), funded by the 5th Framework Programme of the European Commission and coordinated by the University of Surrey, UK – S. Arber and K. Davidson, Work Package 5: What is the role of formal and informal networks in food procurement and consumption in late life?
2 Professor Sara Arber, Mr Tom Daly and Dr Robert Meadows, CRAG, University of Surrey, UK.

References

Arber, S., and Cooper, H. (1999) 'Gender differences in health in later life: The new paradox?', *Social Sciences and Medicine*, 48(1): 61–76.
Arber, S., Davidson, K., and Ginn, J. (2003) 'Changing approaches to gender and later life', in S. Arber, K. Davidson, and J. Ginn (eds), *Gender and Ageing: Changing*

Roles and Relationships (pp. 1–14), Maidenhead: Open University Press/McGraw Hill Education.
Calasanti, C. (2003) 'Masculinities and care work in old age', in S. Arber, K. Davidson, and J. Ginn (eds), *Gender and Ageing: Changing Roles and Relationships* (pp. 15–30), Maidenhead: Open University Press/McGraw Hill Education.
Calasanti, T., and King, N. (2005) 'Firming the floppy penis: Age, class and gender relations in the lives of old men', *Men and Masculinities*, 8(1): 3–13.
Cameron, E., and Bernardes, J. (1998) 'Gender and disadvantage in health: Men's health for a change', *Sociology of Health and Illness*, 20(5): 673–93.
Connell, R. (2000) *The Men and the Boys*, Berkeley, CA: University of California Press.
Courtney, W. H. (1998) 'College men's health: An overview and call to action', *Journal of American College Health*, 46(6): 279–90.
Courtney, W. H. (2000) 'Constructions of masculinity and their influence on men's well-being: A theory of gender and health', *Social Science and Medicine*, 50: 1385–1401.
Davidson, K., and Arber, S. (2003) 'Older men's health: A lifecourse issue?', *Men's Health Journal*, 2(3): 72–5.
Davidson, K., and Meadows, R. (2010) 'Older men's health: The role of marital status and masculinities', in B. Gough and S. Robertson (eds), *Men, Masculinities and Health: Critical Perspectives* (pp. 109–124), London: Palgrave.
Davidson, K., Arber, S., and Ginn, J. (2000) 'Gendered meanings of care work within late life marital relationships', *Canadian Journal on Aging*, 19(4): 536–53.
Emslie, C., Hunt, K., and O'Brien, R. (2004) 'Masculinities in older men: A qualitative study in the west of Scotland', *Journal of Men's Studies*, 12: 207–26.
Giddens, A. (1994) *Modernity and Self-Identity: Self and Society in the Late Modern Age*, Cambridge: Polity Press (orig. 1991).
Goldscheier, F. K. (1990) 'The aging of the gender revolution: What do we know and what do we need to know?', *Research on Aging*, 12: 531–45.
Gough, B. (2006) 'Try to be healthy but don't forgo your masculinity: Deconstructing men's health discourse in the media', *Social Science and Medicine*, 63(9): 2476–88.
Hearn, J. (1995) 'Imaging the aging of men', in M. Featherstone and A. Wernick (eds), *Images of Aging; Cultural Representation of Later Life* (pp. 97–115), London: Routledge.
Jackson, D. (1990) *Unmasking Masculinities: A Critical Autobiography*, London: Unwin Hyman.
Jackson, D. (2003) 'Beyond one-dimentional models of masculinity: A life-course perspective on the processes of becoming masculine', *Auto/Biography*, 11(1–2): 71–87.
Lee, C., and Owens, R. G. (2002) *The Psychology of Men's Health*, Buckingham: Open University Press.
McVittie, C., and Willcock, J. (2006) '"You can't fight windmills": How older men do health, ill health, and masculinities', *Qualitative Health Research*, 16(6): 788–801.
Mason, J. (1996a) *Qualitative researching*, London: Sage.
Mason, J. (1996b) 'Gender, care and sensibility in family and kin relationships', in J. Holland and L. Adkins (eds), *Sex, Sensibility and the Gendered Body* (pp. 15–36), London: Macmillan.

Meadows, R., and Davidson, K. (2006) 'Maintaining manliness in later life: Hegemonic masculinities and emphasized femininities', in T. Calasanti and K. Slevin (eds), *Age Matters: Realigning Feminist Thinking* (pp. 295–311), New York: Routledge.

Moynihan, C. (1998) 'Theories of masculinity', *British Medical Journal*, 317: 1072–5.

Noone, J., and Stephens, C. (2008) 'Men, masculine identities and health care utilisation', *Sociology of Health and Illness*, 30(5): 711–25.

Petersen, A. (1998) *Unmasking the Masculine: 'Men' and 'Identity' in a Sceptical Age*, London: Sage.

Ribeiro, O., and Paul, C. (2008) 'Older male carers and the positive aspects of care', *Ageing and Society*, 28(2): 165–83.

Robertson, S. (2003) 'Men managing health', *Men's Health Journal*, 2(4): 111–13.

Robertson, S. (2006) 'Not living life too much of an excess: Lay men understanding health and well-being', *Health: An Interdisciplinary Journal for the Social Study of Health, Illness and Medicies*, 10: 175–89.

Rose, H., and Bruce, E. (1995) 'Mutual care but differential esteem: Caring between older couples', in S. Arber and J. Ginn (eds), *Connecting Gender and Ageing* (pp. 114–128), Buckingham: Open University Press.

Sabo, D. (2005) 'The study of masculinities and men's health; an overview', in M. Kimmel, J. Hearn, and R. Connell (eds), *Handbook of Studies on Men and Masculinities* (pp. 326–352), London: Sage.

Salisbury, J., and Jackson, D. (1996) *Challenging Macho Values: Practical Ways of Working with Adolescent Boys*, London: Falmer Press

Saltonstall, R. (1993) 'Healthy bodies, social bodies: Men's and women's concepts and practices of health in every day life', *Social Science and Medicine*, 36(1): 7–14.

Segal, L. (1990) *Slow Motion: Changing Masculinities, Changing Men*, London: Virago.

Seidler, V. (1994) *Unreasonable Men*, New York: Routledge.

Solimeo, S. (2008) 'Sex and gender in older adults' experience of Parkinson's disease', *Journal of Gerontology: Series B, Social Sciences*, 63B(1): S42–8.

StatBase (2002). Population: Age, sex and legal marital status, 1971 onwards England and Wales: Population trends 109. Retrieved July 2011, from http://www.statistics.gov.uk/STATBASE/xsdataset.asp?vlnk=5753.

Strauss, A., and Corbin, J. (2008) *Basics of Qualitative Research: Grounded Theory Procedures and Techniques*, 3rd edn, London: Sage.

Thomas, M., Walker, A., Wilmot, A., and Bennet, N. (1998) *Living in Britain: Results from the 1996 General Household Survey*, London: Stationery Office.

Thompson, E. (1994) 'Older men as invisible men', in E. Thompson (ed.), *Older Men's Lives* (pp. 1–21), Thousand Oaks, CA: Sage.

Thompson, E., and Whearty, P. (2004) 'Older men's participation: The importance of masculinity ideology', *Journal of Men's Studies*, 13(1): 5–24.

Victor, C., Scambler, S., Shah, S., Cook, D.G., Harris, T., Rink, K., and de Wilde, S. (2002) 'Has loneliness amongst older people increased? An investigation into variations between cohorts', *Ageing and Society*, 22(5): 585–97.

Watson, J. (2000) *Male Bodies: Health, Culture and Identity*, Buckingham: Open University Press.

White, A. (2001) 'How men respond to illness', *Men's Health Journal*, 1(1): 18–19.

Whitehead, S. (2002) *Men and Masculinities: Key Themes and New Directions*, Cambridge: Polity Press.

11 Aging men, masculinity and Alzheimer's

Caretaking and caregiving in the new millennium

Bethany Coston and Michael Kimmel

America is becoming a caregiving nation. Parents are spending more time with their children than at any other time in our history. Increased longevity means that those same parents are also likely to be providing care, either simultaneously or sequentially, to their own parents as they care for their children. At least 29 percent (65.7 million) of Americans care for either a child or parent (National Alliance for Caregiving and AARP 2009).

Moreover, Alzheimer's is becoming a major concern for the aging population. As the number of people with dementia increases each year, more people than ever will be assuming the roles of caregiver or care-receiver. And while everyone is capable of caregiving and care-receiving, the expectations are different for men and women within these roles. In fact, although currently more women than men provide care or receive care, if present trends continue, the twenty-first century will see many more – perhaps even *most* – men becoming either a giver or recipient of Alzheimer's care. And when they do, they're sure to bump up against traditional notions of masculinity. In this way, we must question, how do men give – and receive – Alzheimer's care? Do they do so differently than women? And, most importantly, do changes in these differences suggest that men in the future may become more effective and nurturing caregivers and more responsive and receptive patients?

To answer these questions we must first start with previous research. Studies have shown that the acceptance of the role of 'patient' varies between men and women. For instance, elderly, disabled and ill relatives rely on the labour of family, with between 50 and 75 percent of all care recipients needing help not only with difficult tasks, such as preparing meals, cleaning the house or managing finances, but also menial ones such as dressing, eating and going to the bathroom (MetLife 2006; Greenwald & Associates 2010).[1] In these ways, being cared for is seen as feminine. To require this kind of care is to be dependent, vulnerable and permeable, contradicting the very tenets of masculinity. This likely accounts for men's higher levels of acting out – swearing, yelling, falling down, making excessive demands and the like – as well as their lower levels of helping behaviours, such as giving praise and helping with caring chores/tasks (Wider 2003).

This is not a surprising response to receiving care. As we know from many scholars, while masculinity varies with both time and place, creating a multitude of masculinities, generally, a dominant model exists – a 'hegemonic' definition of masculinity, to which men are expected to adhere (Connell 1992: 735–51; Connell and Messerschmidt 2005: 829–59; Githens et al. 1994). And in the United States, the dominant image of masculinity that emerged in the nineteenth century was 'the self-made man' (Kimmel 1996). Known generally for manly stoicism and fierce resolve, he was emotionally impenetrable, an armour-plated machine who showed no weakness.

In the mid-1970s, psychologists created a masculinity scale that codified these traits (O'Neil 1981: 61–80), and Brannon and David defined for the field the four basic 'rules' of manhood (1976: 1–48):

1 'No Sissy Stuff': Manhood is defined by distance from what was perceived as feminine.
2 'Be a Big Wheel': Manhood is measured by the size of one's paycheck; wealth, power, status, and success are its defining features.
3 'Be a Sturdy Oak': Manly stoicism is what makes men reliable in a crisis.
4 'Give 'em Hell': Men are adventuresome, exhibiting risk-taking and aggression.

More recently, Kilmartin broke these down into 12 distinctive personality traits: strength, independence, achievement, hard-working, dominance, heterosexuality, toughness, aggressiveness, unemotional, physical, competitiveness, forcefulness (Kilmartin 2000). As we can see, these are not traits that allow much in the way of weakness, reliance or care-receiving. What's more, these traits do not set most men up with adequate caregiving skills. These traditional definitions of masculinity retain a powerful influence over what both men and women believe men should be, and as such, set both men and women up for difficult late-life experiences.

In particular, aging men, aside from the specific conditions of a disease or disability, confront many struggles when faced with diminishing masculinity. Take for instance two personal narratives of men's struggles with caregiving and care-receiving, that of Ted and Harry.[2]

When Ted's wife, Marjorie, was diagnosed with Alzheimer's three years ago at age 73, he was completely unprepared. A 77-year-old retiree, Ted had been slowing down a bit, and filled his days with golf and shopping, watching his beloved Padres on television, and making toys for their five grandchildren who lived in other states. 'I had no idea how to care for Marjorie,' he said.

> What did I know? It was so foreign, like learning another language. I mean, I'm from the generation of men who never changed a diaper for our kids, never cleaned the bathroom, never made the beds. Heck, I can barely fry an egg! But she was losing it – every day, right in front of

me, and I had no idea how to care for her. I sort of panicked. I would sometimes go for long drives, so I wouldn't have to be there. I even started drinking a bit. But then I sort of kicked myself in the butt, and said to myself, 'Ted, you got to play the hand you're dealt.' But I won't tell you it hasn't been hard – or that I didn't look at myself, cleaning yet another soiled sheet, and think 'What a wimp you are, man.'

'Harry had always been so fiercely independent,' his wife Linda said of her 92-year-old husband who'd been diagnosed with Alzheimer's disease four years earlier.

You know, he was the essence of a self-made man. He'd always worked for himself, running his own business, being the family chauffeur, an equal partner in the kitchen. But as his disease progressed, I could see that sense of autonomy and the pride he took in being so independent, slowly eroding. He'd deny it, of course. Try to fight through it. Pretend he understood when he didn't, that he recognized people or remembered events when I knew he didn't. I played along, trying to affirm that sense of himself, even as I knew we couldn't sustain the charade. Gradually, we couldn't any more. He left the stove on a couple of times, and I became afraid he could hurt himself, or just get hurt, or even burn the house down.

Once when I was cooking dinner, I grumbled that I needed a tomato. Harry said, 'I'll get it honey,' and after I protested, he walked to the store. He came back with a potato. I tried not to get angry – he seemed so pleased with himself for running the errand. I said 'A tomato, not a potato.' He looked so embarrassed, sheepish, like a little boy who had displeased his mother. 'I'll go get it,' he said. 'I promise.' How could I not let him go? I wrote '1 tomato' on a piece of note paper, and sent him back to the store, only a block or two away. He came back 20 minutes later and triumphantly presented me with another potato. The note paper was crumpled into a ball in his pocket. He said he had looked at it, but couldn't really remember what it was for.

Ted and Harry represent two sides of the Alzheimer's male equation, patient and caregiver. For sure, the physical or literal act of caregiving and being cared for know no gender. Both women and men are *capable* of caregiving, and both certainly may be in *need* of care. Yet caregiving, and being cared for, are among the most gendered activities in which we engage today.

Women the likely caregivers

Both giving and receiving care is seen as feminine. Caring is an expression of what is often perceived as a 'natural' femininity, an extension of women's biological and evolutionary imperative to care for the young. Caring requires emotional resources as well as various skills, and these emotional resources – patience, calm and nurturance – have, rightly or wrongly, long been coded as 'feminine'.

There is a growing scholarship on the feminization of later life; specifically, the relationship between aging and women. As earlier studies have shown, women are more likely to be caregivers and they make more substantial sacrifices for the role (Arber and Ginn 1993: 33–46). In 2010, of the 11.2 million people in the US caring specifically for Alzheimer's and dementia patients, 7.4 million or two-thirds are women. Female caregivers provide more hours of care and a higher level of care than male caregivers. For example, the new Alzheimer's Association *Women and Alzheimer's* poll[3] shows half of women caregivers and a third of men caregivers are providing more than 40 hours per week of care. Another study shows women spend an average of four hours more caregiving per week than men (22.9 hours for women vs 18.9 hours for men), and female caregivers are more likely than males to help with the personal activities of getting dressed (33 percent vs 24 percent respectively), bathing or showering (30 percent vs 20 percent), and dealing with incontinence or diapers (18 percent vs 13 percent). Moreover, over half of female caregivers of people with Alzheimer's and other dementias are employed, mostly full-time; and 50 percent said they did not have a choice in accepting responsibility for providing Alzheimer's care (Greenwald & Associates 2010; National Alliance for Caregiving and AARP 2009).

Masculinity and the male Alzheimer's patient

Women are more likely the caregivers and men more likely the patients. For women, we see that being a caregiver in late life is often seen and understood as an extension of their caregiving in early and mid-life. It is a role which they should be properly set up for throughout their entire lives. However, being a patient contradicts the very definitions of manhood, leaving a person vulnerable, weakened and dependent.

As a result, many men resist seeking healthcare. Men pay far less attention to diet and substance abuse than women, and they perform self-exams and seek preventive screenings less often as well. Why? As health researcher Will Courtenay writes (Courtenay 1999):

> A man who does gender correctly would be relatively unconcerned about his health and well-being in general. He would see himself as stronger, both physically and emotionally than most women. He would think of himself as independent, not needing to be nurtured by others. He would be unlikely to ask others for help. ... He would face danger fearlessly, take risks frequently, and have little concern for his own safety.

The Alzheimer's Association *Women and Alzheimer's* poll[4] shows a stark gap in the responses of men and women caring for someone with Alzheimer's when asked if they themselves fear developing the disease. Two-thirds of women report they are frightened of developing Alzheimer's; nearly 60 percent of men state they are not. This feeling and acknowledging of health-related vulnerability and fear is one of the largest gender gaps of the poll.

Avoidance of healthcare could also be related to the often-demeaning nature of the medical visit – it is cold, you are naked, and the doctor is talking to you as if you're a child. Others, even, see it as a waste of money – perhaps why more men are uninsured than women. Maybe it's the 'what I don't know can't hurt me' approach. However, the very requirements that make a man a 'real man' may be the very things that endanger his health. The four causes of death that have the highest differential by sex are the four illnesses most closely associated with gender behaviour, not biological sex: accidents, suicide, cirrhosis (drinking) and homicide (Broom and Cavenagh 2010: 869–76). A researcher once suggested creating a warning label: 'Caution: Masculinity May be Hazardous to your Health.'

Alzheimer's can be experienced by men as emasculating: the mind's gradual diminishment may be experienced as a loss of manhood. Caregivers, both male and female, need to be aware of the ways that succumbing to Alzheimer's – indeed, contracting the disease in the first place – can be experienced as gender non-conforming, and that some male patients will attempt to compensate for their perceived loss of manhood by emphasizing other dimensions of that traditional role.

For instance, Alzheimer's may be especially difficult to reconcile with traditional notions of masculinity that stress autonomy and control, because these are often eroded by the disease. This strain is especially present when normal routine activities are compromised. For example, 'the ability to continue driving into late life is germane to factors both intrinsic (related to a sense of self) and extrinsic (a sense of community) that contribute to life satisfaction in old age. Remove this ability, and the loss felt, for men in particular, is deeper than that of simply not being able to get from A to B; it is a loss of a sense of self, of the meaning of manhood' (Davidson 2008: 44–7).

In one study, over half (52 percent) of care recipients had difficulty in carrying out three or more activities of daily living such as bathing, dressing and eating. Nearly nine out of 10 (89 percent) reported difficulty with one or more instrumental activities of daily living (e.g. preparing meals, using the telephone, managing money, taking medication (see Table 11.1) (California Caregiver Resource Centers 2001).

This strain on gender identity experienced by male care recipients may also be the source of some gender differences in patient behaviour. For instance, male Alzheimer's patients may be more likely to act out and less likely to help their caregivers. Care recipients' problematic behaviours have been studied extensively and are consistently found to be influential predictors of caregiver distress (Pinquart and Sörensen 2003: 250–67; Schulz *et al.* 1995: 771–91). Such problems (e.g. falling down, making excessive demands or asking repetitive questions) are typically associated with either physical

Table 11.1 Top functional problems of Alzheimer's care recipients

Functional problem	% reporting problem in previous week
1. Requires supervision of care tasks	75
2. Taking medications	75
3. Managing money or finances	72
4. Staying alone	70
5. Bathing/showering	69
6. Preparing meals	68
7. Performing household chores	67
8. Dressing	65
9. Grooming	55
10. Mobility	55
11. Using the telephone	52
12. Incontinent	48
13. Using the toilet	45
14. Transferring	43
15. Eating	37
16. Wandering	14
Mean no. of functional problems	9

Adapted from: *California CRC Uniform Assessment Database, 2001, N=3,476.*

illness or cognitive impairment (Bookwala and Schulz 2000: 607–16). A recent study discovered that, indeed, wife caregivers reported a higher incidence of problem behaviours among their care-receiving male spouses (Bookwala and Schulz 2000: 607–16).

And these problem behaviours – falling down, questioning, excessive demands, cursing, yelling, and so on – were a significant causal factor in caregiving wives' rates of reported depression. Husbands' problem behaviours can be a significant predictor of wives' maladaptation to caregiving (Seltzer and Li 1996: 614–26). That is, wife caregivers whose husbands exhibited problem behaviours were likely to feel distant from their husbands and burdened by caregiving. Despite this, it is important to note that men who live alone have been shown to have poorer health than those who live with a partner. 'Marital status is a key factor, with lone older men lacking the skills to establish and maintain social networks and particularly likely to be socially excluded' (Davidson and Arber 2004:127–48). It has been argued that the needs of the aging male patient population require urgent consideration (Davidson *et al.* 2003: 168–85).

Masculinity and the male Alzheimer's caregiver

The same things that make a male patient feel emasculated often make being a male caregiver stressful and make it difficult to incorporate the role responsibilities into the traditional definitions of masculinity. However, it's important to remember that just because men may perform caregiving differently from women it doesn't necessarily mean they do it worse.

Male caregivers, for example, tend to believe that they can simply 'add' caregiving to their list of other activities. Male caregivers are more likely to be working full-time (60 percent) than female caregivers (41 percent), and female caregivers are more likely to be working part-time (14 percent) than male caregivers (6 percent) (Greenwald & Associates 2010). However, this could be because women were more likely than men to have decreased their hours, passed up promotions or assignments, took leaves of absence, switched their employment from full- to part-time, quit jobs or retired early because of their caregiving role.

In another study, conformity to traditional masculinity was actually associated with having greater perceived competence at caregiving (Wilken et al. 1996: 37–42). After all, while caring may be gender-nonconforming, being good at what you do (competence) may be an even stronger masculine-gendered trait. However, it's equally clear that such an additive model of caregiving, in which the caregiver simply adds the caregiving duties to an otherwise long list of gender-conforming activities, can also be quite stressful for the caregiver. One California study found that being a caregiver for Alzheimer's patients is associated with increased risk for cardiovascular disease, especially for males (Mills et al. 2009: 605–10).

Outside of an additive model, we see that traditional masculinity ill prepares men for traditional caregiving – as mentioned prior, the traits associated with masculinity do not leave much, if any, room for nurturing tendencies. However, unlike women caregivers of men patients, who struggle with their husband's problem behaviours and obstinacy, husbands may feel less depression than women in caregiving positions because they receive *help* from their wives in the caregiving process. Miller reported that female care recipients provided their caregiving spouses with several forms of support, which included helping with chores, providing companionship and making them feel useful (Miller 1990: 311–21). These helping behaviours can lessen the stress of caregiving. Indeed, Kaye and Applegate (1993) found that male caregivers in general described emotional gratification as an important motivation for caregiving.

Overall, it seems as though women caregivers are more greatly affected psychologically and physically by caring for an Alzheimer's patient (Greenwald & Associates 2010). However, we must keep in mind that the tenets of masculinity call for stoicism and being unemotional, both of which would lead men to underreport or not report their feelings of stress, depression or pain from the job.

Caring and receiving care in the twenty-first century

Caregiving is not an 'identity', something you are, but rather a set of practices, something you 'do'. While gender shapes our experiences of both the giving and the receiving of care, it is equally true that anyone – male or female – can be an effective caregiver. In fact, in the past two decades, men have increased the amount of time they spend in caregiving with their young children enormously. Men now spend as much time with children in 2010 as women did in 1980. (Women have also increased their time!)

Men have increased their caregiving with children at little cost to their sense of themselves as men. And if men can do it with their children, it's possible that they can also become more active and involved with their parents and spouses. And if that is possible, then it is even possible that they can receive care in ways they had not previously.

The current cohort of men who are both Alzheimer's patients and caregivers are also from an earlier era, likely born before the advent of the gender revolution of the 1960s. More likely to subscribe to more traditional gender identities, this is a generation that may be inhibited by the gender roles of the past. They are men like Harry, who prided himself on his autonomy and independence in the public sphere, and men like Ted who seemed equally proud of his 'dependence' in the private sphere – that is, his learned helplessness, his inability to take care of himself – as a badge of masculinity.

Younger cohorts of men are more egalitarian at home and at work. They are as accustomed to female colleagues and co-workers as they are competent at cooking and cleaning. As these men age, the traditional ideologies to which their fathers and grandfathers subscribed will be, at least partly, supplanted by a masculinity of nurturance, caregiving and love. And they will, hopefully, feel no less manly for it.

Notes

1 Access to unpublished data made possible by Maria Shriver and the Alzheimer's Association in conjunction with Geiger *et al.* (2010).
2 This information comes from interviews conducted by Michael Kimmel.
3 Poll and data available in Geiger *et al.* (2010).
4 Ibid.

References

Arber, S., and Ginn, J. (1993) 'Gender and inequalities in health in later life', *Social Science and Medicine,* 36: 33–46.
Bookwala, J., and Schulz, R. (2000) 'A comparison of primary stressors, secondary stressors, and depressive symptoms between elderly caregiving husbands and wives: The caregiver health effects study', *Psychology and Aging,* 15: 607–16.
Brannon, R., and David, D. (1976) 'The male sex role: Our culture's blueprint of manhood, and what it's done for us lately', in R. Brannon and D. David (eds), *The Forty-Nine Percent Majority: The Male Sex Role,* Boston, MA: Addison-Wesley.

Broom, A., and Cavenagh, J. (2010) 'Moralities, masculinities and caring for the dying: An exploration of experiences of living and dying in a hospice', *Social Science and Medicine*, 71: 869–76.
California Caregiver Resource Centers (2001) Uniform Assessment Database: http://www.caregiver.org/jsp/content_node.jsp?nodeid=1040.
Connell, R. W. (1992) 'A very straight gay: Masculinity, homosexual experience, and the dynamics of gender', *American Sociological Review*, 57: 735–51.
Connell, R. W., and Messerschmidt, J. W. (2005) 'Hegemonic masculinity', *Gender and Society*, 19: 829–59.
Courtenay, W. H. (1999) 'Better to die than cry? A longitudinal and constructionist study of masculinity and the health risk behavior of young American men' (Doctoral dissertation, University of California at Berkeley), *Dissertation Abstracts International*, 59(08A): 232pp. (publication number AAT 9902042).
Davidson, K. (2008) 'Declining health and competencies: Older men facing choices about driving cessation', *Generations*, 32: 44–7.
Davidson, K. and Arber, S. (2004) 'Older men: Their health behaviours and partnership status', in A. Walker and C. Hagan Hennessey (eds), *Growing Older: Quality of Life in Old Age* (pp. 127–48), Maidenhead: McGraw-Hill.
Davidson, K., Daly, T., and Arber, S. (2003) 'Exploring the worlds of older men', in S. Arber, K. Davidson, and J. Ginn (eds) *Gender and Ageing: Changing Roles and Relationships* (pp. 168–185), Maidenhead: Open University Press/McGraw Hill.
Geiger, A. T., Morgan, O., Meyer, K., and Skelton, K. (eds) (2010) *The Shriver Report: A Woman's Nation Takes on Alzheimer's*, New York: Free Press/Simon & Schuster.
Githens, M., Norris, P., and Lovenduski, J. (1994) *Different Roles, Different Voices: Women and Politics in the United States and Europe*, New York: Harpercollins College Division.
Greenwald, M., & Associates. (2010) Unpublished data from the NAC/AARP survey of caregiving in the US, prepared under contract for the Alzheimer's Association.
Kaye, L. W., and Applegate, J. S. (1993) 'Family support groups for male caregivers: Benefits of participation', *Journal of Gerontological Social Work*, 20: 167–85.
Kilmartin, C. (2000) *The Masculine Self*, New York: McGraw-Hill Humanities/Social Sciences/Languages.
Kimmel, M. S. (1996) *Manhood in America*, New York: Free Press.
MetLife (2006)*The MetLife Study of Alzheimer's Disease: The Caregiving Experience:* http://www.metlife.com/assets/cao/mmi/publications/studies/mmi-alzheimers-disease-caregiving-experience-study.pdf.
Miller, B. (1990) 'Gender differences in spouse caregiver strain: Socialization and role explanations', *Journal of Marriage and the Family*, 52: 311–21.
Mills, P. J., Ancoli-Israel, S., Mausbach, B. T., Aschbacher, K., Patterson, T. L., Ziegler, M. G., Dimsdale, J. E., and Grant, I. (2009) 'Effects of gender and dementia severity on Alzheimer's disease caregivers' sleep and biomarkers of coagulation and inflammation', *Brain, Behavior, and Immunity*, 23: 605–10.
National Alliance for Caregiving and AARP (2009) *Caregiving in the U.S: 2009*. MetLife Foundation: http://www.caregiving.org/data/Caregiving_in_the_US_2009_full_report.pdf.
O'Neil, J. M. (1981) 'Male sex role conflicts, sexism, and masculinity: Psychological implications for men, women, and the counseling psychologist', *The Counseling Psychologist*, 9: 61–80.

Pinquart, M., and Sörensen, S. (2003) 'Differences between caregivers and noncaregivers in psychological health and physical health: A meta-analysis', *Psychology and Aging*, 18: 250–67.
Schulz, R., O'Brien, A. T., Bookwala, J., and Fleissner, K. (1995) 'Psychiatric and physical morbidity effects of dementia caregiving: Prevalence, correlates, and causes', *The Gerontologist*, 35: 771–91.
Seltzer, M. M., and Li, L. W. (1996) 'The transitions of caregiving: Subjective and objective definitions', *The Gerontologist*, 36: 614–26.
Wider, J. (2003) 'Alzheimer cases expected to skyrocket over next fifty years', *Society for Women's Health Research*: http://www.womenshealthresearch.org/site/News2?page=NewsArticle&id=5399&news_iv_ctrl=0&abbr=press.
Wilken, C. S., Altergott, K., and Sandberg, J. (1996) 'Spouses' self-perceptions as caregivers: The influence of feminine and masculine sex-role orientation on caring for confused and non-confused partners', *American Journal of Alzheimer's Disease and Other Dementias*, 11: 37–42.

Index

Abbott Laboratories 35
abuse 106
active sensibility 186
active surveillance (AS) 62n6
ADAM *see* androgen deficiency in the aging male
adaptation 90, 99, 156, 177; Atchley's theory of 89
Afghanistan, war in 77
ageism 1, 25, 54, 90, 112, 140
agency 6, 7, 22, 26, 30 *see also* autonomy; lack of 31, 32
aging delay 1–2 *see also* anti-aging medicine/technologies
The Aging Male 41
AIDS 108, 110, 111
Akkus, Professor 162, 164
Akşam 161
Albanian migrants in rural Australia 95, 97, 99
alcohol consumption 23, 176, 180, 187
Altman, Dennis 108
Alza Corporation 39
Alzheimer's disease: caregiving 191–8; de-masculinization 195; and HRT 41; masculinity and the male Alzheimer's caregiver 197; masculinity and the male Alzheimer's patient 194–6; top functional problems of care recipients 196 Tbl.
American College of Physicians 37
Androcur 117n4
Androderm 40
AndroGel 35, 44–5, 46, 49n3
androgen deficiency in the aging male (ADAM) 36, 43, 45, 78, 79 *see also* testosterone-deficiency syndrome (TDS); Third Age; PADAM (partial androgen deficiency in the aging male) 43, 47
androgen replacement therapy 38, 40, 47, 78–80; testosterone 29, 35–6, 37–40, 41, 42, 44–7, 48, 78–80
androgen suppressants 117n4
andropause 5, 11–12, 13, 29, 35–48, 157; as affront 166; and the crisis of masculinity in the 1990s 36–9; definitions 159–60; as an excuse for marital infidelity 164–6; and the female menopause *see* menopause; framed as a health problem 161–4; and late-onset hypogonadism 45–6, 48; and low testosterone levels 35–6, 37–8, 42–4; and masculinities 36–9, 156, 159–60 *see also* masculine identity/masculinities; as mid-life crisis 161, 162–4, 165, 166; pharmaceuticalization 35–48, 157, 160 *see also* anti-aging medicine/technologies; biomedicine/biomedicalization; medicalization; and sexuality *see* de-masculinization; sexuality; testosterone; and testosterone replacement therapy 29, 35–6, 37–40, 41, 42, 44–7, 48, 78–80; in Turkey 156–67; and Viagra 40–2 *see also* Viagra
Annals of Long Term Care 38
anti-aging medicine/technologies 2, 28, 29, 32, 49n2, 110, 111, 112, 113, 117, 138, 140–51 *see also* biomedicine/biomedicalization; medicalization; and new aging 112–14, 116
anti-aging practices 22, 26, 27, 29, 32
anti-war movement 76

anxiety 10, 25, 58, 87, 110; about aging, in Turkey 11, 157, 161, 162, 163, 164, 165, 166, 167
arthritis 148
Atasoy, Attila 161
Atchley, R. 89
Australia, CALD migrants *see* migrant men from CALD backgrounds in rural Australia
autonomy 22, 179, 193, 195, 198 *see also* agency; independence; migrants of CALD backgrounds in later life maintaining identity and 91–101
Auxilium Pharmaceuticals 45
Ayalan, Sukru 166
azgın teke syndrome 161, 164–6, 167

baby boomer generation 25, 26
back pain, chronic low-back 148
Barrett, C. 115, 117n4; *et al.* 115
Basting, A. D. 26
Bauer, M. *et al.* 106
Bauman, Z. 24, 25, 26
Beck, U. 21, 24
Bengston, V. L. *et al.* 89
biomarkers 2
biomedicine/biomedicalization 1–2, 4–5, 9, 13, 56, 73, 107 *see also* anti-aging medicine/technologies; medicalization; challenge to biomedical perspective on aging 86–101; and erectile dysfunction 79–80, 81, 123–4, 125–6, 129–30, 134–5 *see also* Viagra; and gay older men 110–12; globalized 14; and the HIV/AIDS epidemic 110, 111, 117n3; and new aging 112–14, 116; and prostate cancer 55–6, 57, 59–61; reproductive biotechnologies 114; sexual performance enhancing drugs 107 *see also* Viagra; and Yoruba men 11, 141, 147–51
Bly, Robert 37
body/embodiment 2, 5, 7, 21–32, 78, 159; consumer society, generation and the older body 24–7; cultural embeddedness of mental health and masculinity 76–8; embodied femininity 74 *see also* femininity; gay male body 106, 110, 111–12; gay older men and the body image 110–11; idealized male body 23; identity tied to the body 52, 55, 56, 61; and the invisibility of older men 31, 53, 60, 87, 113; Leder on the body 52; masculinity, youthfulness and the body 22–4, 25, 27, 28–30, 42; and medicalization *see* anti-aging medicine/technologies; biomedicine/biomedicalization; medicalization; normalization of the male body 5; postmodern body 25–6; prostate cancer and the aging body 53–61; 'resexing' of aged body 28; sexual body 28, 55–7, 80 *see also* testosterone; sexuality *see* sexuality; shift of impotence from mind to body 40–1, 78; social body 59–60; statistical body (body at risk) 57–9; Turkish male body 159; youthful male body 23, 27 *see also* youthfulness
Bove, R. and Valeggia, C. 139, 149
'brain training' 31
Brannon, R. and David, D. 192
Broom, A. and Tovey, P. 2
Brown, P. *et al.* 74

Calasanti, C. 185
Calasanti, T. 24–5, 27; and King, N. 28; and Slevin, K. 26
CALD (culturally and linguistically diverse) men in rural Australia *see* migrant men from CALD backgrounds in rural Australia
Cameron, E. and Bernardes, J. 176
caregivers: Alzheimer's 191, 193–4, 195–8; female 193–4, 197; male 160, 194, 197; service providers 100–1, 115; Yoruba 146, 150, 151; for young children 198
Carruthers, M. 38–9, 42, 43
choice 7, 26
Cialis 28
civil rights movement 76
Clarke, A. E. *et al.* 5, 73, 81
compliance 140, 182–3
Connell, R. W. 2, 108, 167–8n1, 189; and Messerschmidt, J. V. 167–8n1
Conrad, P. 5, 72, 157
consumer culture/lifestyle 22–3, 24–7, 28; commercial gay culture 108, 110–11, 112, 113–14; and identity 113–14
consumption 7, 22, 25, 26, 27, 29, 30; alcohol 23, 176, 180, 187

continuity 92, 99, 177; Atchley's theory of 89; discontinuity 92
control 10 *see also* agency; autonomy; of the body through lifestyle 25, 181
cosmetics 27, 111, 112, 113; cosmetic surgery 22, 29, 107
Courtenay, W. H. 176, 194
cultural beliefs 96, 140–1
cultural identity: of CALD men in rural Australia 92–4, 97–9; as men, and medicalization 71–82
culturally and linguistically diverse men in rural Australia *see* migrant men from CALD backgrounds in rural Australia

Davidson, K. *et al.* 185
de-masculinization 9, 13, 27–8, 31, 54, 72, 81, 115, 160, 177; and Alzheimer's 195; and prostatectomy 56; testosterone, andropause and 36, 42, 45
depression 37, 43, 77, 140, 162–3, 196
DHEA (Gynodian Depot) 54
diagnostic testing 55–6, 57–8, 59, 60–1
discrimination 106, 109, 112, 115, 116, 150 *see also* ageism
Duman, S. 161
Duncan, D. 112–13
Duru, Nükhet 168n6

ED *see* erectile dysfunction
Ellis, A. and Abarbanel, A. 107
embodiment *see* body/embodiment
Endocrine Society 45
Endocrinology and Metabolism Clinics 38
enhancement drugs 2, 107 *see also* Viagra
erectile dysfunction (ED) 5, 11, 13, 56, 72, 81; decreasing erectile function in Mexico 123–35; global discourse and local difference 125–6; and medicalization 79–80, 81, 123–4, 125–6, 129–30, 134–5 *see also* Viagra; post-surgical 56; and Viagra 40–2
Ersan, M. 162
European Association of Urology 47

fake drugs 148, 150

Falkland War 77
families: and Alzheimer's 192–4, 196, 197; role with migrant men from CALD backgrounds in rural Australia 94–6, 98–100
fatigue 35, 42, 43, 76
Featherstone, M. 26
femininity 27, 42, 74, 76, 81, 116, 139, 179, 193; and homosexuality 111
feminism 8, 52, 105, 158, 186; feminist scholarship 4, 71, 72–3, 91, 105, 157, 168n4, 188; second wave 188
Finley, E. P. 77
Fishman, J. R. 41, 78
Fourcroy, Jean L. 40
Fourth Age 1, 8, 22, 32; negotiation of 30–1; Third Age/Fourth Age distinction 6–7, 54
Fox, N. J. and Ward, K. J. 75
Fredriksen-Goldsen, K. and Muraco, A. 108, 109

gay culture 105; commercial 108, 110–11, 112, 113–14; queer subcultures 108
gay liberation 108, 111
gay masculinity 108
gay older men 105–17, 159; abuse of 106; biomedicine, body image and 110–12; and care settings 115–16; discrimination against 106, 109, 112, 115, 116; and exceptionalism 105–7, 116–17; and healthy aging 111–14; and medical fictions 107–8; and prostate cancer 117n3; and research literature 105, 106–9; and stereotypes of homosexuality 107, 115–16
gender: and the body *see* body/embodiment; and the compromise of men's health 37, 38–9, 55–6, 100–1, 105; feminism *see* feminism; gendered approach to aging 90–1, 176; gendered power relations 2, 139, 149; and healthy aging 86–101; identity *see* identity; masculine identity/masculinities; and migration 86–101; and post-structural theory 5; research on intersection of health and 160; theory 2
Geriatrics 38

Giddens, A. 184–5
Gilleard, C. and Higgs, P. 6, 22, 26, 27, 30–1
globalization 14, 125, 141, 158
Gough, B. 176
Gulf War Syndrome (GWS) 76–7, 81
Gynodian Depot (DHEA) 54

HAART (highly active antiretroviral therapies) 110, 117n3
Haber, D. 109
hair transplants 5
Harman, S. M. 47
Hartley, H. 29
Hattat, Halim 163
health care 175–88; Alzheimer's care 191–8; being cared for seen as feminine 191, 193; beyond biomedicine and institutional care, challenge of CALD migrants 100–1; caregivers *see* caregivers; caring and receiving care in the twenty-first century 198; gender and the compromise of men's health 37, 38–9, 55–6, 100–1, 105; medicalized *see* biomedicine/biomedicalization; medicalization; men and health professionals 38–9, 177, 182–4; older gay men and care settings 115–16; paradox of older men and caring 175, 176, 184–7; service providers 100–1, 115 *see also* caregivers
healthy aging 88–92; among the Yoruba 146–7; challenge to biomedical perspective on aging 86–101; of gay men 111–14; life-course perspective on 96–101; migrant men in rural Australia 86–8, 92–101; and the role of the family 94–6, 98–100; and sexual activity 106–7, 112, 113
Hearn, J. 31
hegemonic masculinities 2, 5–6, 13, 23, 32, 73, 156, 160, 167–8n1, 176; diminishing need for 24; and lifestyles 160; and machismo *see* machismo; in Turkey 159–67
hetero-normative sexuality 2, 5, 13; privileging of 105–7, 116–17
Higgs, P. and Jones, I. R. 22
highly active antiretroviral therapies (HAART) 110, 117n3
Himcaps 126

Hirschfeld, M. 54
HIV 108, 110, 115, 117n3, 139
Hockey, J. and James, A. 28
homophobia 10, 55
homosexuality: and exceptionalism 105–7, 116–17; and femininity 111; gay liberation 108, 111; gay masculinity 108; and the HIV/AIDS epidemic 110, 111, 115, 117n3; homosexual culture *see* gay culture; homosexual older men *see* gay older men; and medical fictions 107–8; stereotypes of 107, 115–16
honour 95, 159
hormone replacement therapy (HRT) 29, 35–6, 37–40, 41, 42, 44–7, 48, 54, 56, 78–80
Hughes, M. 107–8
Hürriyet 161, 162, 163, 164
hypogonadism 39–40, 45, 46, 162; late-onset (LOH) 45–6, 48

idealized masculinity 1, 10, 21, 28, 55, 86 *see also* hegemonic masculinities; idealized male body 23
identity: and the commercial scene 113–14; cultural *see* cultural identity; masculine *see* masculine identity/masculinities; migrants of CALD backgrounds in later life maintaining autonomy and 91–101; and ontological security 184–5; and sexual performance 8, 123, 144, 162–3, 167; tied to the body 52, 55, 56, 61; and work 97–8
impotence 29, 35, 40–2, 55, 56, 78 *see also* erectile dysfunction (ED)
IMSS (Instituto Méxicano del Seguro Social) 126–30, 135
independence 1, 10, 31, 96, 192, 198 *see also* autonomy
individualization 7
industrialization 23–4
infidelity, marital 12, 146, 149, 161, 164–6, 167
Institute of Medicine (IOM) 46–7
Instituto Méxicano del Seguro Social (IMSS) 126–30, 135
International Society for the Study of the Aging Male (ISSAM) 1, 41, 44, 45, 47
invisibility, of older men 31, 53, 60, 87, 113

in vitro fertilisation (IVF) 114
IOM (Institute of Medicine) 46–7
Iraq, war in 77
irritability 35, 42, 43, 76, 162–3
Islam 166
ISSAM (International Society for the Study of the Aging Male) 1, 41, 44, 45, 47
Italian migrants in rural Australia 92–3, 95
IVF 114

Jackson, D. 177, 186
Jones, I. R. and Higgs, P. 25, 26
Jones, J. and Pugh, S. 27, 112
Journal of Andrology 79
Journal of Clinical Epidemiology 38
Journal of Men's Health 79

Karner, T. X. 74
Kartal, A. 163
Katz, S. and Marshall, B. L. 44, 114, 116
Kaye, L. W. and Applegate, J. S. 197
Kelly, J. 108
Kilmartin, C. 192
Kilshaw, S. 76, 81
Kolankaya, Aytug 168n3
Korean War 74, 75
Köseli, B. 165
Krafft-Ebbing, Richard von 107
Kunar, S. 165

late-onset hypogonadism (LOH) 45–6, 48
Leder, D. 52
libido 35, 42, 43, 54, 76, 131, 140, 144, 160, 162–3, 164
Liek, E. 53
life-course perspective on healthy aging 96–101
lifestyles: consumer *see* consumer culture/lifestyle; control of the body through 25, 181; Fourth Age 31 *see also* Fourth Age; male 23, 24, 112–13, 160, 180–1; of older gay men 112–13; reckless 146–7; self-reliant 1; Third Age 1, 27, 30 *see also* Third Age; Yoruba 140, 146–7
Loe, M. 28
LOH (late-onset hypogonadism) 45–6, 48
Lunenfield, B. 41

McDonald, L. 88–9
Macedonian migrants in rural Australia 94, 96, 97–9
machismo 10–11, 37, 38–9, 42, 123, 124, 133, 134, 177; and problematic youthful sexuality 130–2
McVittie, C. and Willcock, J. 177
male climacteric 36, 43, 162 *see also* andropause
male lifestyles 23, 24, 112–13, 160 *see also* lifestyles
male menopause *see* andropause
marginalization of older men 53, 54–5, 87, 114, 156; gay men 105, 109
marital infidelity 12, 146, 149, 161, 164–6, 167
Marshall, B. L. 42, 45, 78, 157
masculine identity/masculinities 8, 10, 12, 23, 24, 25, 30, 156, 177, 183, 185, 186, 188; age-appropriate masculinities 123–35; and andropause 36–9, 156, 159–60 *see also* andropause; and the body *see* body/embodiment; Brannon and David's four basic rules of manhood 192; commodification of 111, 160 *see also* consumer culture/lifestyle; crisis in the 1990s 36–9; cultural beliefs, medicine use and 140–1; gay masculinity 108 *see also* gay older men; homosexuality; health, aging and 176–8, 180–1 *see also* prostate cancer; hegemonic *see* hegemonic masculinities; idealized *see* idealized masculinity; identity and sexual performance 8, 123, 144, 162–3, 167; loss of 162; and machismo *see* machismo; and the male Alzheimer's caregiver 197; and the male Alzheimer's patient 194–6; and medicalization *see* anti-aging medicine/technologies; biomedicine/biomedicalization; medicalization; Mexican *see* Mexican masculinities; migrants of CALD background maintaining identity and autonomy in later life 91–101; multiple masculinities 176; and polygyny 138–40, 149, 150 *see also* Yoruba; and the resistance of femininity 74, 76, 81, 179; the self-made man 192; and

sexuality *see* sexuality; sexualized 27, 29, 55, 115; and stoicism 91, 175, 177, 182, 192, 197; and testosterone *see* testosterone; Turkish *see* Turks; and war 73–80, 81–2; of the Yoruba 140–51
Mason, J. 186
Mathar, T. and Jansen, Y. 6
medicalization 4–5, 30, 71–82, 157, 160 *see also* anti-aging medicine/technologies; biomedicine/biomedicalization; and addiction fears 147–8; cultural beliefs, masculinity and medicine use 140–1; endorsing and resisting, in combat-related mental health problems 77–8; and erectile dysfunction 79–80, 81, 123–4, 125–6, 129–30, 134–5; fake drugs 148, 150; men's health and theory and interpretations of 72–3; process comparisons, PTSD and TDS 80–2; self-medication 147, 148; TDS, ED and endorsement of 78–80; testosterone and the pharmaceuticalization of male aging 35–48; in Turkey 157; of veteran's health symptoms 74–7, 81–2; war, mental health, masculinity and 73–80, 81–2; and Yoruba men 11, 141, 147–51
menopause 11, 12, 36, 37, 41, 43, 157, 159, 163–4, 167; male *see* andropause
men's health movement 105, 117n2
men's movement 37
mental health: and the accumulation of stressful events 87; healthy aging *see* healthy aging; PTSD *see* post-traumatic stress disorder; war, masculinity, medicalization and 73–8, 81–2
Mexican masculinities 123–35; and decreasing erectile function 123–35; and ideals of changing sexuality across the male life course 132–4; machismo 123, 124, 130–2, 133, 134; and problematic youthful sexuality 130–2; stereotypic masculinities and local complexities 134–5; and understandings of health, aging and ED drugs 128–30
mid-life crisis 161, 162–4, 165, 166 *see also* andropause

migrant men from CALD backgrounds in rural Australia 86–8, 92–101; and the challenge to health care beyond biomedicine and institutional care 100–1; and the concept of healthy aging 89–90; cultural identity 92–4; family role 94–6, 98–100; gendered approach 90–1; life-course perspective 96–101
Mild Cognitive Impairment (MCI) 31
Milliyet 161, 166
Miner, M. M. 79–80
Minichiello, V. *et al.* 32
Mol, A. and Law, L. 52–3
Mosse, G. L. 75
Moynihan, C. 176–7
Muftuoglu, O. 163–4, 165

National Agency for Food and Drug Administration and Control (NAFDAC, Nigeria) 150, 151
National Cancer Institute (NCI) 46
National Institute of Aging (NIA) 46
National Men's Health Policy (Australia) 86–7
NCI (National Cancer Institute) 46
Neco 168n6
neoliberalism 1
new aging 112–14, 116
NIA (National Institute of Aging) 46
Nigeria, Yoruba 11, 140–51
Noone, J. and Stephens, C. 183

obesity 23
oestrogen 37, 46, 56
ontological security 184–5
Orwoll, E. S. 38
osteoporosis 37, 38, 41, 157
Öztürk, Yasar Nuri 165

partial androgen deficiency in the aging male (PADAM) 43, 47
Paz, O. 131
Pfizer 40
pharmaceuticalization 35–48, 72–3 *see also* medicalization
pink economy 111
polygyny 149; and masculinities 138–40 *see also* Yoruba; polygynous sexuality 138–51
postmodern body 25–6
post-structural theory 5
post-traumatic stress disorder (PTSD) 72, 74, 75–8; comparison of

medicalization in TDS and 80–2; and GWS 76–7
Potts, A. *et al.* 150–1
power relations, gendered 2, 139, 149
Powersex 126
Premarin 37
prostate cancer 52–61; and the aging body 53–4; and biomedicine 56, 57, 59–61; of gay men 117n3; PSA test 57–9; risk 57–9; self-support groups 59; and the sexual body 55–7; and the social environment 59–60
prostatectomy 56
prostate gland 55, 164; cancer of *see* prostate cancer
PSA test 57–9
PTSD *see* post-traumatic stress disorder

queer theorists 105–6

reductionism, medical 48
reflexive modernization 21
regrets 140, 188
Reiger, K. 94
'Reinardo' 59
religious faith 97
re-masculinization 76; testosterone as agent of 45, 47 *see also* testosterone: replacement therapy
reproductive biotechnologies 114
Republican People's Party (RPP, Turkey) 166
resilience 92, 109, 175
retirement 28; mandatory 24
Roberts, C. 29
Robertson, S. 2, 176, 181, 187
Robinson, P. 112, 113
Rose, H. and Bruce, E. 186
Rose, N. 2, 5, 58
Rosenberg, C. 48
Rosenfeld, D. 106–7; and Faircloth, C. A. 2
Rubin, G. 114
Ryan, G. W. and Bernard, H. R. 143

Sabah 161
Sabo, D. 160; and Gordon, D. F. 2
Salamone, F. 149
Scheper-Hughes, N. and Lock, M. 52–3
Scherrer, K. S. 106
Schwaiger, E. 25
second modernity theories 7, 21

security, ontological 184–5
Seidler, V. 177
self-medication 147, 148
sentient activity 186
sexual body 28, 55–7, 80 *see also* testosterone
sexual dysfunctions 9, 29, 35, 47, 48, 86; erectile *see* erectile dysfunction (ED)
sexuality 27–8; African sexualities 141 *see also* Yoruba; and the andropause *see* andropause; de-masculinization; testosterone; and arthritis 148; and cultural ageism 1; de-sexualization/de-masculinization *see* de-masculinization; and the embodied self 57; gay *see* gay older men; homosexuality; healthy aging and sexual activity 106–7, 112, 113; hetero-normative *see* hetero-normative sexuality; homosexuality *see* gay older men; homosexuality; identity and sexual performance 8, 123, 144, 162–3, 167; libido *see* libido; and low-back pain 148; macho 123, 124, 130–2, 133, 134 *see also* machismo; marginalized forms 139; marital infidelity 12, 146, 149, 161, 164–6, 167; masculinity, sexuality and growing older 27–30; and medicalization *see* anti-aging medicine/technologies; biomedicine/biomedicalization; medicalization; Mexican ideals of changing sexuality across the male life course 132–4; performance enhancing drugs 2, 107 *see also* Viagra; polygynous 138–51; 'resexing' of aging bodies 28; sex-role theory 71; sexual activity of older men 54, 106–7, 112, 113, 132 *see also* Viagra; sexual desire *see* libido; sexualized masculine identity 27, 29, 55, 115; and society 123–35, 138–51; and testosterone *see* testosterone; in Turkey 158; women's 145, 150–1; of the Yoruba 140–51; youthful 28, 29, 30, 113, 129, 130–2, 134
shame 127, 140, 157, 160, 167, 168n2

shell-shock 75 *see also* post-traumatic stress disorder (PTSD)
smoking 23, 176, 180–1, 187
social body 59–60
Solimeo, S. 177
Solvay Pharmaceuticals 35, 44
statistical body (body at risk) 57–9
Stengel, R. 37
stoicism 91, 175, 177, 182, 192, 197
surrogacy 114

TDS *see* testosterone-deficiency syndrome
Tenover, J. L. 38
Testim 45, 46
Testoderm 39–40
TestoGel 44, 49n3
testosterone 5, 29; Institute of Medicine report 46–7; 'Low T' 35, 37–8, 42–4 *see also* androgen deficiency in the aging male (ADAM); andropause; testosterone-deficiency syndrome (TDS); measurement of levels 43, 48; patch 39–40; and the pharmaceuticalization of male aging 35–48; replacement therapy 29, 35–6, 37–40, 41, 42, 44–7, 48, 78–80
testosterone-deficiency syndrome (TDS) 72; comparison of medicalization in PTSD and 80–2; and endorsement of medicalization 78–80
Theratech 40
Third Age 1, 8, 22, 24, 26, 27, 28, 29–30, 32; negotiation of 30, 31; Third Age/Fourth Age distinction 6–7, 54
Thompson, E. H. 31, 177
Toplum and Bilim 158
Toprak, Halis 165
Torres, S. 89, 92, 96
Traish, A. M. *et al.* 79
Turgut, S. 166
Turks 156–67; andropause discourses in Turkey 161–7; migrants in rural Australia 93, 96, 97, 99–100, 151; the 'new Turkish man' 158; research on Turkish masculinities 158–9

Unimed Pharmaceuticals 44
urbanization 23–4

van den Hoonaard, D. B. 3
Viagra 5, 28, 40–2, 48, 55, 79, 80, 81, 107, 125, 134, 151, 157
Vietnam War 75–6, 77
Visser, R. O. *et al.* 30
Von Gyurkovechky, V. G. V. 55

war 73–80, 81–2
watchful waiting (WW) 58, 62n6
Watkins, E. S. 37
Watson, J. 23
Weksler, M. E. 38
WHI (Women's Health Initiative) 46
White, A. 183
Whitehead, S. M. 23
Willison, K. and Andrews, G. 139
Women and Alzheimer's 194–5
Women's Health Initiative (WHI) 46
women's health movement 71, 105
women's movement 76
work, and identity 97–8
World Health Day (2012) 1
World Health Organization 151
World War II 75

Yassin, A. A. and Saad, F. 79
Yoruba 140–51; and masculinity 11, 140–51; and medicalization 11, 141, 147–51; socio-demographic profile of interviewees 143, 144Tbl., 145Tbl.
Young, A. 76
youthfulness 23, 25, 27, 28–30, 42; youth culture 22, 26, 27; youthful sexuality 28, 29, 30, 113, 129, 130–2, 134

Zaman 161, 165–6

Taylor & Francis
eBooks
FOR LIBRARIES

ORDER YOUR FREE 30 DAY INSTITUTIONAL TRIAL TODAY!

Over 23,000 eBook titles in the Humanities, Social Sciences, STM and Law from some of the world's leading imprints.

Choose from a range of subject packages or create your own!

Benefits for you
- Free MARC records
- COUNTER-compliant usage statistics
- Flexible purchase and pricing options

Benefits for your user
- Off-site, anytime access via Athens or referring URL
- Print or copy pages or chapters
- Full content search
- Bookmark, highlight and annotate text
- Access to thousands of pages of quality research at the click of a button

For more information, pricing enquiries or to order a free trial, contact your local online sales team.

UK and Rest of World: **online.sales@tandf.co.uk**
US, Canada and Latin America: **e-reference@taylorandfrancis.com**

www.ebooksubscriptions.com

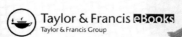

A flexible and dynamic resource for teaching, learning and research.